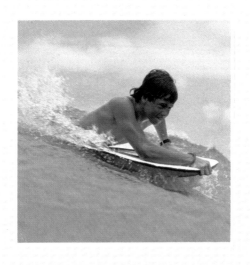

A FAMILY GUIDE TO HEALTHY LIVING

FITNESS & EXERCISE

DR. GORDON JACKSON

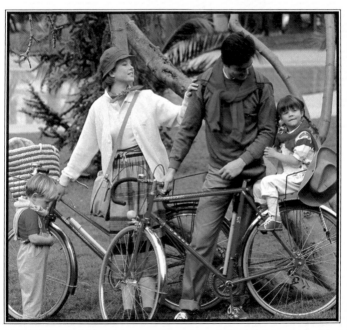

TAFELBERG

Originally published by
Salamander Books, London
© 1985 Salamander Books
South African English edition
© 1989 Tafelberg Publishers Ltd,
28 Wale Street, Cape Town 8001

ISBN 0 624 02835 6

AUTHOR

Dr Gordon Jackson qualified in medicine from Cambridge University
and Guy's Hospital Medical School in 1971. Since then he has followed
a career in internal medicine, and is now a consultant physician
on the staff of Lewisham Hospital and Guy's Hospital Medical
School. Dr Jackson specialised in heart conditions early in his
career, but later broadened his interest to include diabetes
and other related diseases. He has researched into the use of
applied physiology in the study of diseases of the heart and
circulation, and is particularly concerned with the effects
of physical exercise and diet. Dr Jackson has written extensively
for the general public on a wide range of medical topics, often in
collaboration with his wife, a family doctor. He is an experienced
marathon runner and long-distance walker, and has developed a
keen interest in water sports.

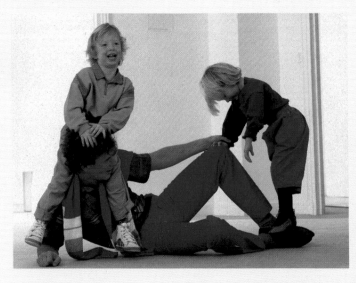

Designer: Kathy Gummer
Picture research: Vickie Walters
Set by Hirt & Carter (Pty) Ltd
First edition, first impression 1989

Colour reproductions:
Rodney Howe Ltd.
Printed in Belgium by Proost
International Book Production.

CONTENTS

INTRODUCTION

Since the middle 1970s there has been a surge of interest in physical fitness. People are suddenly beginning to shake off their lethargy and get themselves fit. Why do they bother? It is quite an effort getting fit and then staying that way – is it really worth all the sweat? Do the fitness fanatics believe they will live longer because of their efforts?

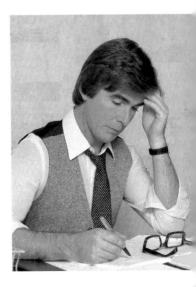

There is a simple answer to all these questions. The reason why thousands of people have got themselves very much fitter than they were before, and have taken the trouble to stay that way, is simply because they feel very much better as a result. Physical fitness makes you feel mentally sharper, physically more comfortable and more in tune with your body, and better able to cope with the demands that everyday life makes upon you. One of the interesting things about the new army of physically fit individuals is how few of them let their fitness slip away again. The reason for this is simple: they simply feel bad if they let themselves slide back into the inactive, unfit lives that they were leading before.

There is only one way of finding out if you too would feel better and enjoy life more if you were fit, and that is to get fit and see how you like it. It would be a pity if you let yourself be put off. Perhaps the most important thing to be aware of is that there are all sorts of ways of getting fit and staying fit. If the idea of putting on your running shoes and going out on to the roads for a long jogging session does not appeal to you, there are many other things that you can do instead. This book explores a wide variety of physical activities – you are sure to find

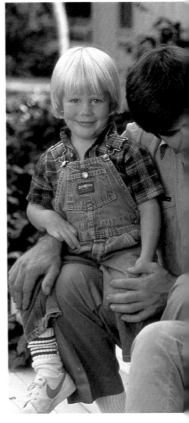

> *Increased physical fitness not only improves health but improves your performance at work. Hundreds of American companies have backed this idea financially by employing full-time directors of fitness for their workforces.*

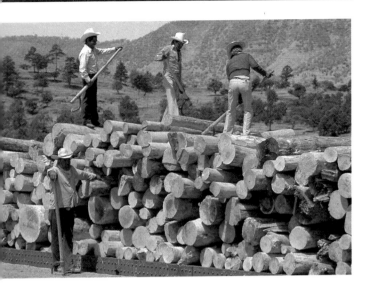

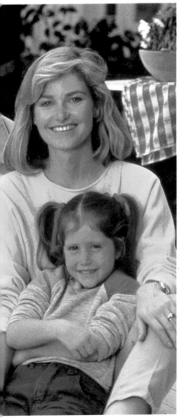

Above left: *Work often involves very little physical exertion these days, and it is easy to become completely sedentary.*
Above: *Some occupations can be as physically demanding as many competitive sports.*
Left: *Settling down to family life may mean an end to regular sport, and a decline in fitness.*

something that appeals to you.

For most people who leave school or college and go into a sedentary job, the end of full-time education also means the end of any sort of sport or physical training. Despite the growth in interest in sport and fitness over the last few years, it remains the case that most of us have given up sport or any other physically strenuous activity by the time we are in our late twenties. The important thing to realize is that it is never too late to start getting yourself fit again. If you are older it will take longer, but it is not necessarily harder; in fact the older you are, the easier you may find it to stick to a plan and achieve your goal. Different approaches may be needed at different ages, however, so we will look at ways of becoming and keeping fit at all stages of life.

DOES FITNESS PROLONG LIFE?

The main cause of death in the western world is disease of the heart and arterial system – the diseases that give rise to strokes and heart attacks. Most people living in developed countries will die of heart or artery disease; deaths from the next biggest killer – cancer – are a lot less common. If physical fitness is to prolong life, therefore, it must prevent heart and artery disease, or at least delay the onset of such problems.

There have been many claims that fitness has been 'scientifically proven' to prolong life. Unfortunately this is not so. There is a lot of scientific evidence on the subject, but it does not add up to what a conscientious scientist would regard as proof. However, it is quite fair to say that there is more evidence in favour of the idea that fitness and exercise make you live longer than there is against.

One of the earliest pieces of evidence came from London, where Professor Morris carried out a study on the drivers and conductors of London double-

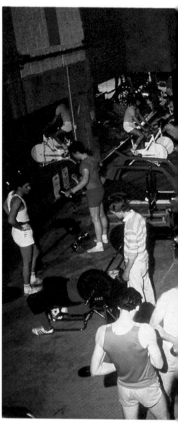

Below: *The conductors of London buses enjoy better health than their drivers, whose occupation is both stressful and sedentary.*

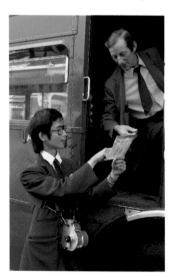

decker buses. It was found that the drivers – who had a rather sedentary occupation – were actually much more at risk from heart problems than the conductors who spent much of their working day exercising by running up and down the stairs of the buses. Since then Professor Morris has produced another study of male civil servants in London, which suggests that those who do most physical exercise in their leisure time are least likely to suffer from heart problems.

There have been many similar studies. Two of the most notable were carried out in the USA by Professor Paffenbarger; one in a population of San Francisco dockers, and the other among graduates of Harvard University.

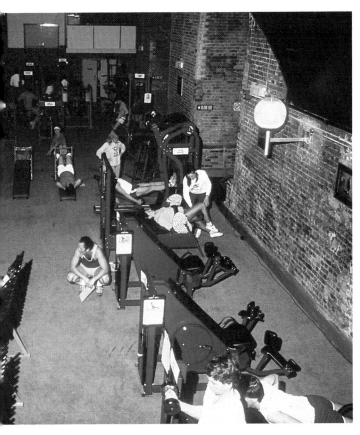

Again both studies suggest that the more you exercise – whether at work like the dockers, or in leisure time like the Harvard graduates – the less risk you run of premature heart and artery disease.

So the case in favour of exercise looks encouraging, but it cannot be regarded as proven. It is possible, after all, that exercise causes as many problems as it prevents. People certainly can die during the course of physical exercise, and many reports of such deaths have reached the newspapers – although this is probably because such deaths are newsworthy whereas improved well-being as a result of exercise is not. Nevertheless it is very important to be sensible about physical training to minimize the risk of any problems developing.

Above: For the city-dweller a gym is an excellent place to work out. Studies of office workers indicate that spare-time exercise reduces the risk of premature heart problems.

Many people say that exercise makes them feel better and more relaxed, and a number of studies have shown that people improve psychologically as well as physically as a result of running programmes. There is a lot of circumstantial evidence to suggest that this relaxing effect is caused by the release of endorphins – morphine-like substances which occur naturally in the brain.

WHAT IS FITNESS?

To appreciate the benefits of fitness you don't need to be trained up to the level of a competitive athlete, and once you have got yourself fit it does not take much effort to stay that way – three or four sessions a week of less than half an hour each are probably all that you need. However, there are considerable differences between activities so far as their value in achieving fitness is concerned. They vary both in the amount of exercise they involve, and in the effect of that exercise. When choosing a basic activity for a fitness programme it is important to understand what is meant by the term 'fitness', and especially what is meant by the term 'aerobic fitness'.

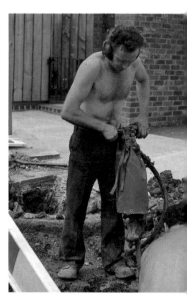

Strength, stamina and flexibility

For someone who has a very heavy job, such as a manual labourer or a forester, the main thing he wants from his body is the strength to carry out all the strenuous tasks that his everyday work involves, and the stamina to keep at them for several hours at a time. Strength and stamina are not the only things that matter though. For someone like a dancer the most important thing is to maintain flexibility and suppleness.

The achievement of total fitness depends upon combining these three main strands: strength, stamina and flexibility. However, it seems that the main benefits to health and well-being are obtained by improving the body's stamina.

The capacity to keep up high levels of physical activity for ever-increasing periods of time is

Above right: *Heavy work demands strength and stamina, which are normally developed in the course of the job. Work like this is particularly good for improving arm and shoulder strength.*
Right: *A supple body is essential for a dancer, but she also needs the stamina to keep going. In everyday life both qualities are equally important.*

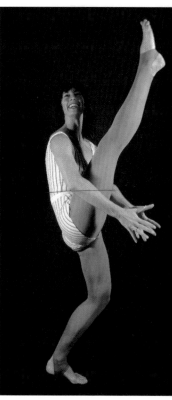

the most obvious benefit of physical training. This capacity depends on a lot more than the individual muscles doing the work. The muscles have to be supplied with the nutrients and oxygen that they need to produce the energy they are expending. All this energy production depends as much upon improving the performance of the heart, the lungs and the bloodstream as upon improving the muscles themselves, and this is what training for stamina achieves.

Aerobic fitness

The whole system which carries oxygen from the air through to the muscles has been called 'the aerobic system', and for this reason training the system for stamina is called aerobic training. Since the heart and the lungs are essential to all the other organs of

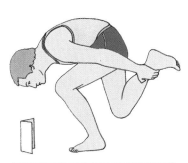

A simple trick to test balance and flexibility: Fold a piece of paper and stand it up on the floor. It should be about 12in (30cm) tall. Stand behind it on one foot, holding the other foot up behind your back. Then pick the paper up in your teeth, if you find this easy, try the other foot!

PHYSICAL FITNESS

There is no single measure of physical fitness, and no single way of achieving it. However, there are three major qualities which contribute to overall fitness:

Strength

Training for physical strength depends upon building up muscle bulk by repeated work with heavy loads.

Stamina/aerobic fitness

Endurance depends as much on the lungs, heart and blood vessels as upon the working muscles themselves. Training which is aimed at improving endurance and stamina is called aerobic training.

Flexibility

It is quite possible to have considerable strength and stamina but to have a body that is very stiff and inflexible. Flexibility is as much a part of overall fitness as strength and stamina.

the body, not just the muscles, improvement in the function of the heart and lungs by aerobic training produces an overall improvement in health and well-being. If aerobic training really does tend to prolong life, then this is likely to be the result of the beneficial effects of exercise on the lungs, heart and circulatory system.

Most people find that aerobic training inevitably carries with it some increase in muscular strength, but unless you are an enthusiastic body-builder there seems very little point in pursuing this aspect of fitness further. There is certainly no direct evidence that putting on ever-increasing amounts of muscle is of any benefit in terms of health or longevity.

Flexibility is a different matter. Some forms of physical training – especially running – lead to some loss of flexibility owing to the tendency of the trained muscles to shorten slightly. Flexibility is very important in everyday life and it is essential to maintain it by appropriate exercises. The 'warm down' exercises described on pages 26-27 have been devised for just this purpose.

You have to use energy to move anything; this rule applies as much to the human body as to any other machine. The energy to move your body comes from the action of your muscles, so your muscles are creating and expending energy with every movement you make.

Muscles use very much the same process to create energy as that used in the engine of a car. In the engine fuel is burnt to produce energy. Oxygen from the air is essential to this process, and the fuel for a car engine is mixed with air before it is burnt. As a result of the combustion of fuel and oxygen, energy is liberated. There are waste products in the form of water and carbon dioxide gas.

Clearly the muscles don't use petrol. Instead they use fuel derived from food – most commonly in the form of sugar. It is combined with oxygen in a sophisticated series of chemical reactions inside the muscle cells. The end result is exactly the same in the muscles as it is in the engine – fuel combustion produces energy, with water and carbon dioxide as waste products.

There are obvious differences of course. In the car engine the energy is released immediately in the form of a controlled explosion. Human cells are a lot more subtle than this.

They are able to store the energy in the form of a chemical called ATP. The stored energy can then be released from the ATP in a controlled manner. It is rather like the wind chest of an organ, or the bag of a set of bagpipes, where the energy is stored up and released at just the right rate by the player. Organs and bagpipes soon run down if there isn't a constant supply of air, and so do muscles if there isn't a constant supply of food and oxygen, but the extra storage step allows them to produce a smooth and controlled action.

If the muscles are going to produce a steady supply of energy by burning up fuel with oxygen, they obviously need a steady supply of these materials delivered to them. In fact it is the delivery of oxygen rather than fuel which is most important, and this is brought about by the combined action of the heart and lungs.

If you are exercising hard, then a lot of muscles are being used. This means that oxygen is being consumed at tissue level at an extraordinarily high rate. A fit athlete of around 76 kg in weight, exercising to his full capacity, may burn up five litres of oxygen every minute. Now oxygen only makes up about a fifth of the atmosphere,

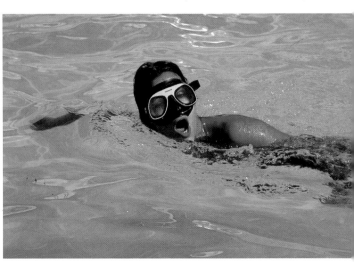

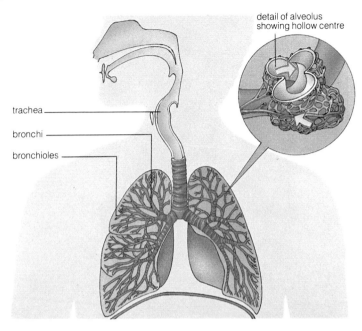

detail of alveolus
showing hollow centre

trachea

bronchi

bronchioles

Above: *The lungs are composed of millions of air sacs called alveoli, connected to the trachea [windpipe] by branching bronchi and bronchioles. Each alveolus is surrounded by blood vessels which absorb oxygen from the air.*
Below left: *A good oxygen supply is essential when exercising hard.*

The purpose of the many tiny air-sacs in the lungs is to provide a big surface area so that oxygen can cross into the blood. In an adult this area is about $65m^2$ – equivalent to half a singles' tennis court.

and the lungs don't extract all the oxygen from it, so to maintain this sort of oxygen delivery to the tissues our athlete may need to inhale approximately 150 litres of air every minute.

Once absorbed through the lungs oxygen must be transported to the tissues via the bloodstream, and this means that the heart may need to pump massive quantities of blood. In fact during heavy exertion it may pump more than 35 litres every minute in a fit person – not bad for an organ the size of two fists clenched together. In contrast the same person at rest would be pumping only four or five litres of blood a minute.

The reason why endurance training is called aerobic training now becomes obvious, since its most important effect is to improve the way that oxygen is carried from the air to the muscles. There is no doubt that aerobic training improves the way in which the heart and lungs work. Compared with an unfit individual, an aerobically fit person will be much less breathless at the same level of exertion, and will have a lower pulse rate too.

The lungs
The first stage in the complex business of getting oxygen from the air to the exercising muscles happens in the lungs. The lungs consist of millions of tiny air sacs, all of which are closely surrounded by blood vessels. These air sacs (the alveoli) are connected to the nose

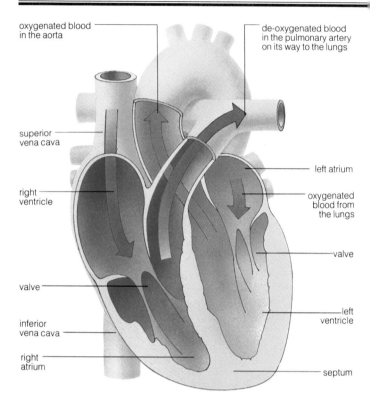

oxygenated blood in the aorta

de-oxygenated blood in the pulmonary artery on its way to the lungs

superior vena cava

left atrium

right ventricle

oxygenated blood from the lungs

valve

valve

left ventricle

inferior vena cava

right atrium

septum

and the mouth by a branching series of tubes – the bronchi. As you breathe, oxygen-rich air is drawn down through the bronchi into the alveoli.

Once the air has reached the alveoli, the blood in the network of tiny vessels which surrounds each of them is able to absorb the oxygen. It then becomes the business of the heart and the circulation to make sure that this oxygen – which is actually carried in the red blood cells – is transported to the exercising tissues. Blood returning from the tissues carries the waste gas carbon dioxide, and this is allowed to escape from the blood into the alveoli and then on out into the atmosphere as you breathe out.

The lungs are really like bellows, sucking air in and then blowing it out again. All the work of this sucking and blowing is done by the muscles of the chest wall which

Above: *De-oxygenated blood from the tissues enters the right atrium of the heart and is pumped to the lungs by the right ventricle. The blood oxygenated in the lungs returns to the left atrium and is pumped out to the tissues via the aorta.*

expand and contract the rib cage, and by the diaphragm – a muscular sheet separating the chest from the abdomen.

The circulation
Blood is always in motion within the circulation, pumped by the heart. Oxygen-rich blood leaving the lungs returns to the heart where it is pumped out through the arteries to all the tissues, including exercising muscles. During exercise, in fact, there is a tendency for blood flow to be diverted towards the exercising muscles and away from other tissues.

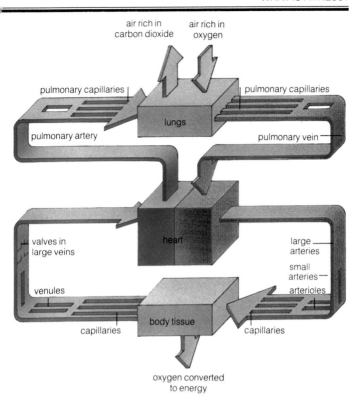

air rich in carbon dioxide

air rich in oxygen

pulmonary capillaries

pulmonary capillaries

lungs

pulmonary artery

pulmonary vein

valves in large veins

heart

large arteries

small arteries

venules

arterioles

capillaries

body tissue

capillaries

oxygen converted to energy

Above: *Oxygen in the lungs is absorbed into the blood, which is pumped to the body tissues by the heart. There the oxygen is used to create energy, and replaced by waste carbon dioxide. The blood then returns to the heart and is pumped back to the lungs.*

Just as the blood is able to accept oxygen from the lungs, so it is able to give it up to the tissues. As the oxygen is lost to the tissues, the blood picks up the waste gas carbon dioxide. The blood then returns via the veins to the heart and thence to the lungs again.

The action of the heart is central to the way in which the circulation works. The heart is a muscle, and it is the action of its muscular walls which produces the pressure to pump blood around the circulation. Blood returns from the tissues at relatively low pressures, and enters the right side of the heart where it is pumped through to the lungs. Enriched with oxygen, the blood returns from the lungs to the left side of the heart. From here the blood has to be pumped around the whole body – not just the lungs – and the pressures need to be much greater. The main pumping chamber which is responsible for this high-pressure pumping is the left ventricle, and its walls are correspondingly thicker than the walls of the rest of the heart.

The effect exercise has on burning up kilojoules is complex, but it certainly speeds up the process. It is said that you continue to burn double the normal number of kilojoules for two hours after a brisk two-hour walk. If you run for half an hour this increase in kilojoule burning may go on as long as six hours.

17

It is possible to carry out very specific tests which measure the amount of oxygen that your body is capable of burning up over the course of a few minutes' hard exercise, while the pulse rate and other aspects of the heart's performance are measured electrically. The few questions and the simple test on this page cannot rival the accuracy of this type of fitness assessment, but they will give an approximate picture of the level at which you function, and an idea of whether you need to get fitter.

A simple fitness test

This test makes use of an ordinary flight of stairs to give a rough assessment of fitness. It depends on taking your pulse after exercise. Find your pulse on the inside of your wrist on the thumb side, and learn to feel it with the two middle fingers of the opposite hand. Count the number of beats in half a minute, and double this number to get the pulse rate.

Be sure your flight of stairs has more than ten and less than twenty steps. Start going up and down the stairs at a good rate – as a guide you should be climbing between three and four steps every two seconds, and running down again. By the end of three minutes you will be quite breathless.

In Canada a thorough enquiry into the sporting habits of the population showed that between 1972 and 1976 the number of Canadians who ran regularly increased by 150 per cent. There was an equivalent increase in the number of regular skiers. The best evidence available from the USA suggests that between 1960 and 1980 the number of adults involved in regular sport doubled.

As with all aerobic activity you should stop at once if you feel uncomfortably breathless, dizzy or faint, or if you get a pain in the chest.

After three minutes stop and wait *exactly half a minute* then time your pulse over the *next* half minute. If your pulse rate is less than 80 per minute you are very fit. If it is over 80, but less than 92 you are probably in quite good shape. If it is over 100 you really need to be fitter. (You can add five beats per minute to these figures if you are female and two beats for every decade over the age of 40).

Below: *Almost every aspect of heart and lung performance is monitored as this athlete works on a bicycle ergonometer.*

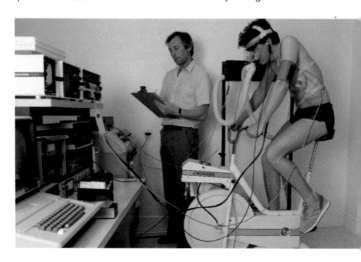

FITNESS QUESTIONNAIRE

Have you walked more than
8 km, or run more than
5 km, or cycled more than
13 km, or swum for more than
20 minutes.

a three times or more within
the last week
b once or twice in the last
week
c within the last month
d or is it more than a month
since you have done any of
these things?

If you have to go up two flights of
stairs and there is a lift
available, do you

a never take the lift and
run up
b walk or run up most of the
time
c use the lift most of the time
d never walk up unless the lift
is actually broken?

You want to visit the shops
which are more than a kilometre
away. Bearing in mind that you
are not pressed for time, would
you

a always walk or bike

b walk or bike if it is a nice day
c drive or go by bus nine times
out of ten
d try and avoid going at all if
someone else could go for you?

How fast would you normally
cover 3 km on fairly flat
ground?
(If you don't know the answer to
this, take a walk and find out)

a in less than 20 minutes,
running
b in less than half an hour at a
brisk walk
c in more than half an hour but
less than 40 minutes
d either you wouldn't even
attempt it or it would take you
longer than 40 minutes

Score

3 for each **a**
2 for each **b**
1 for each **c**
0 for each **d**

Add up the total, then see below
for an assessment of your fitness.

11-12
You are quite likely to be fit, and
you could be very fit. If you want
to improve your fitness further it
is simply a question of building
up your exercise levels. There is
no need to take any special
precautions.

8-10
You are probably reasonably fit,
but you may be beginning to slip
below the level of exercise which
is desirable from the health point
of view. It would do you no harm
to step up your exercise levels a
bit, but make sure you are not at
risk (see page 32).

4-7
You almost certainly have a way
of life which does not provide
the exercise levels which are
recommended for health. It is
highly desirable to get fitter, but
you should proceed with
caution, especially if you are
over 35 (see page 30).

0-3
You are either very unfit or very
young. Either way it is time to get
fitter, but *proceed with caution*.
If you do too much too soon
you are very likely to suffer some
injury, which may be serious
(see page 30).

MUSCLES AND JOINTS

All the work of movement is done by the muscles. These work by shortening, so they are only capable of pulling, not pushing. Two-way movement is achieved by two sets of muscles, which pull in opposing directions.

An individual muscle is attached at each end to bone. There is invariably a joint in between the points of attachment, so as the muscle shortens the joint moves. Sometimes the point of attachment is a long way from the main body of the muscle, in which case the connection is made by a tendon – a tough cord of fibrous tissue.

Muscle structure
Muscles are actually bundles of fibres. Within each fibre there are smaller, parallel fibres, and these are the source of muscle contraction. When the nervous system signals the muscle to contract, the small parallel fibres slide past each other, telescoping to shorten the muscle.

The fibres which make up muscle are not all the same. Some of them – known as fast twitch fibres – respond to the stimulus to contract very quickly and very forcefully. Others – the slow twitch fibres – are slower to respond. Obviously there has to be some advantage in having the slow twitch fibres, otherwise we would all have the more responsive fast twitch

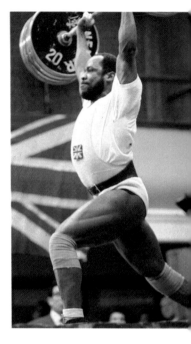

Above: *Explosive sports such as weightlifting or sprinting depend on the fast twitch muscle fibres. These work anaerobically, and do not rely on the delivery of oxygen from the lungs and heart.*
Below: *When a muscle contracts, the fibres slide together to reduce its length. On relaxation they slide apart again.*

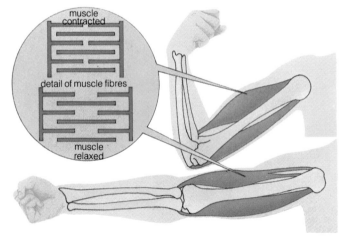

muscle contracted

detail of muscle fibres

muscle relaxed

variety in all our muscles. In fact it is the slow twitch fibres which bear the brunt of any prolonged exertion. They will keep working for hours whereas the fast twitch fibres are there for sudden explosive effort.

The proportion of the two different types of fibre in the muscles varies from person to person. Among top class sportsmen, endurance athletes such as long distance runners and cyclists have mostly slow twitch fibres in their muscles. In contrast sprinters, throwers and weightlifters have a predominance of the fast twitch 'explosive' fibres.

Slow twitch fibres work by continuously converting oxygen and sugar into energy. They need a steady supply of oxygen, so endurance athletes have to breathe regularly and deeply throughout the competition.

Fast twitch fibres work by storing up large amounts of energy in the form of the high energy chemical bonds which make up ATP. The energy can then be released on demand to produce muscular effort. These fibres don't use oxygen while they are working, but work solely on stored energy. However, a lot of oxygen will be needed after the sudden effort is over, to make good the energy they have used. This is known as the 'oxygen debt'. A graphic example

> *When a muscle contracts, most of the energy produced from the burning fuel is wasted as heat, and only 30 per cent is actually converted into mechanical work. However, the heat production is vital for warm-blooded animals as it maintains body temperature.*

is the hundred-metre sprinter, who may take only one or two small breaths during the race but will still be puffing for a half a minute or so after. Clearly this sort of muscle activity is not very useful over a long distance.

Aerobic training primarily works on the slow twitch fibres, increasing the efficiency with which they can turn oxygen and fuel into energy. A number of interesting things happen during this training. For example, it has been suggested that the slow twitch fibres begin to run better on different fuels – not just on sugar. The fuel they turn to is in fact fat, which may explain why aerobic exercise has such a dramatic effect in helping some people to lose weight.

Below: *Marathon running is one of the most aerobically demanding of sports. It depends mainly on the action of the slow twitch muscle fibres.*

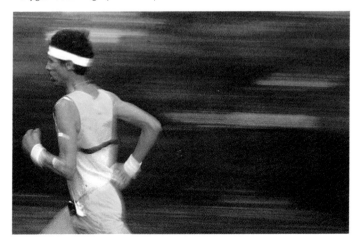

The skeleton

Your body depends upon its skeleton. Without it you would collapse into a shapeless lump of jelly. It is no good having a rigid skeleton, however, if you lose mobility as a result, so most of the bones are connected by a system of joints.

The joints in the body each have different functions and different ranges of movement. In the leg, for example, the hip joint has to be able to move in almost all directions, so it has a ball and socket arrangement. The knee only needs to move in one basic direction, like a hinge. The mass of small bones and joints which make up the ankle and foot provide flexibility coupled with stability, because although the joints between each small bone can move, none of them can move far.

The situation is much the same in the arm, although the joints are less robust since they do not have to bear the weight of the body. There is a mass of small joints in the hand, a hinge joint at the elbow and a multi-dimensional ball and socket joint at the shoulder.

How joints work

All the joints in the body have the same basic components. A layer of cartilage covers the surface of each bone where it rubs against the other. Lubrication for these surfaces is provided by synovial fluid, and the whole mechanism is contained within a 'joint capsule'.

Most types of arthritis result from a failure of the lubrication system. There is some evidence that frequently putting all the joints through their full range of movement

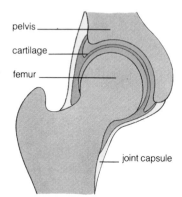

pelvis

cartilage

femur

joint capsule

Above: *The ball and socket joint at the hip is padded with cartilage and lubricated by the synovial fluid contained within the joint capsule.*

helps to ward off those forms of arthritis that are due to wear and tear. Exercise of all sorts will help.

A joint needs stability as well as lubrication, otherwise it would soon pull itself apart. This stability is provided by a series of ligaments around each joint which run between the two connecting bones in the directions where the joint is put under most strain. The ligaments are sheets or cords of fibrous tissue, just like the muscle tendons.

The muscles which act on the joint also provide a lot of physical stability, and you can certainly strengthen joints by strengthening the muscles around them.

Injury

Any of these structures can be injured. Most of us think that bone fractures are the most serious type

Above: *With age, joints become less mobile, and this may lead to arthritis in later life. Most of the joints are kept flexible*

by other forms of exercise, but the neck joints will benefit from being regularly put throuth the full range of movements.

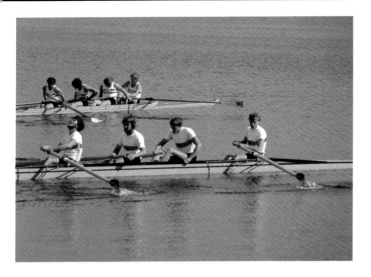

Above: *Strenuous sports such as rowing put the muscle-joint system under considerable strain which can result in injury. Proper training and warm-up precautions are essential.*

of injury, and in many ways this is so. However, a straightforward fracture may heal a lot quicker than some injuries to ligaments; serious damage to a ligament may lead to permanent loss of function in the joint concerned.

Injuries in contact sports are clearly unavoidable, but many other sporting injuries are brought about by over-exertion and failure to take sensible precautions. Most people tend to forget to warm up properly, and then push themselves too hard, especially as they are starting out on the road to fitness.

The risk of injury to muscles and joints increases if very similar movements are repeated time and time again. For this reason it is a good idea to change the terrain that you run over. When running on tracks and roads, the surface is never even and one foot is always hitting the ground a fraction earlier than the other – it is usually the foot nearer the middle of the road. Be sure to cross the road from time to time or run in the opposite direction, and this will spread the load. It is also well worth varying the nature of the surfaces you run over. Grass makes a change from tarmac or concrete, and may prove easier on the feet.

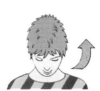

Above: *The neck roll exercise involves rolling the head back, sideways, forward and round, and repeating ten times. Do this every day, but do it gently. As with all exercises, too much enthusiasm can cause strains which may take weeks to heal.*

The purpose of aerobic exercise is to improve the function of the individual muscles, and the performance of the heart, blood vessels and lungs which supply them with the oxygen they need. However, there is no point in doing this if all your efforts result in repeated muscle and joint injuries.

There is no doubt that by increasing your level of sporting activity you inevitably increase

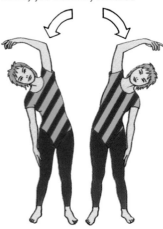

the risk of injury, especially to the joints, muscles and tendons, but this risk can be kept to a minimum if you take precautions. The most important of these is to make sure your muscles warm up progressively before you indulge in really heavy exertion.

The reason why warming up is so essential is simple. When you are at rest, the rate of blood flow to the muscles is quite low, but during vigorous exercise it is very high. If you go straight from rest into a period of really hard physical exertion the level of blood flow will not have time to catch up. The function of the muscles will be impaired, and in this state they are easily overstressed. This is the time when injuries occur. On the other hand, if you start off gently and wait until the level of blood flow is adequate in the warmed-up tissues, you are much less likely to suffer from injuries such as pulled and strained muscles.

Warming up can take many different forms. You can just set out doing your normal aerobic exercise at a lower intensity, or you may find it easier to start off with some gently warm-up exercises before you start working hard. It doesn't matter how you let your muscles work up to their high-level blood flow, as long as you give them the chance to do so. If you don't you are very likely to run into trouble, and you may have to give up training for some time.

Above: *Waist Stretch. Swing from side to side from the waist, but try to keep your hips still.*
Below: *Toe Touch. Stand straight with your arms raised, then bend your knees and let your arms swing through behind you, then swing back upright again.*

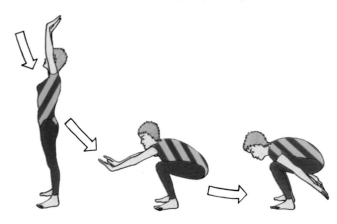

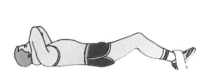 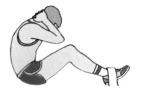

Above: *Sit-Ups. Initially it is easier to do sit-ups with your knees bent and your feet hooked under something to give you more* leverage. *As you improve you can straighten your legs. This exercise is designed to strengthen the abdominal muscles.*

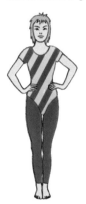 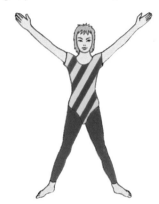 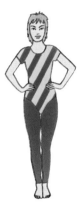

Above: *Stride Jumps. This is an excellent way to warm up and encourage the blood flow. Start with your feet together, then* spring to an astride position, then spring back to your original posture. Start gently: about one complete jump per second.

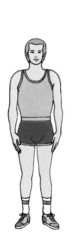 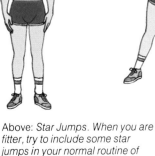 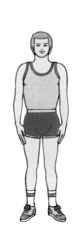

Above: *Star Jumps. When you are fitter, try to include some star jumps in your normal routine of exercise. Start with your feet* close together, then jump up and make the star illustrated in the middle drawing, then land with your feet close together again.

25

'Warming down' is important for runners, and others who are involved in a sport which is predominantly running (or walking) and does not involve much in the way of stretching.

The problem with running, which is otherwise an excellent and convenient form of aerobic exercise, is that it tends to *reduce* rather than increase flexibility. When you are running, the same groups of muscles are in use all the time, and they go through the same range of movements with each step that you take. Over the course of time this leads to some shortening of the muscle fibres. If the muscles themselves are shorter it inevitably reduces the range of movement in the joints which they control. Runners tend to shorten the hamstrings at the back of the thighs, thus limiting their capacity to bend forward at the hips. They also shorten the calf muscles, and this restricts ankle movement.

Fortunately these problems are easy to get over, provided that you put these muscles on a bit of stretch at the end of your training. The curiously named 'warming down' exercises on this page are designed to do just this.

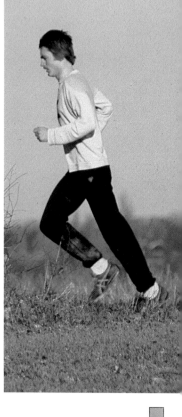

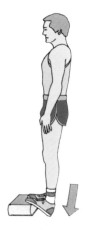

Above: *Kerb Drop. Stand on the edge of a kerb; as you drop your heels, you will feel your calves stretching.* Don't bounce. *Repeat gently five times.*

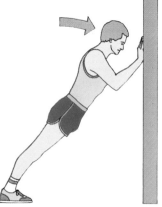

Above: *Wall Stretch. Stand at arm's length from a wall, then bend your arms and lean forward. Like Kerb Drop, this will stretch you Achilles tendons.*

Achilles tendinitis, inflammation of the thick cord-like tendon at the back of the heel, is the commonest of runners' injuries – with as many as 15 per cent of a sample of 900 long-distance runners suffering from it severely enough to stop training. Court-game players are also at risk. Gentle stretching of the tendon during the 'warm-down' period goes a long way towards preventing trouble.

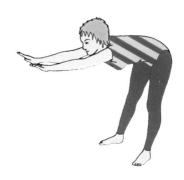

Left: *At the end of a run it is important to do some muscle-stretching 'warm down' exercises.* Below: *Roll-Overs. Stretch out on the floor, then bring your legs as far over your head as you can. Not for those with back problems.*

Above: *Hamstring Stretch. Start with your feet apart, and bend over forwards keeping your knees locked straight. It is important to keep your back hollowed. As you bend, you will feel the backs of your thighs stretching.*

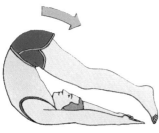

Right: *Thigh Shift. Extend one leg sideways and then bend the opposite knee. You will feel your inner thigh stretch. Repeat five times for each leg. Don't bounce.*

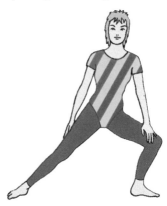

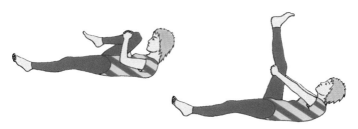

Above: *Knee Hugs. Lie down, and hug your knee as closely as possible to your chest while keeping the other leg straight. This stretches the hamstring.*

Above: *Leg Pulls. Keeping your leg straight and your foot relaxed, pull your knee towards your head. Then point your toes down towards your face.*

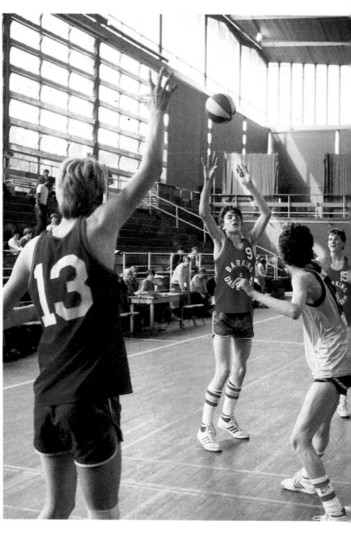

Above: *Before embarking on any really strenuous exercise such as a competitive basketball game, it is essential to minimize the risk of injury by ensuring all your muscles are well warmed up, either by a series of exercises (see pages 24 and 25) or by a gentle warm-up phase of the game. This will stimulate the blood flow to the tissues and ensure it is adequate to cope with the demands made by your muscles during the game itself.*

Warming up is much more important in cold weather than at other times. The body shuts down blood vessels to stop heat loss, and this increases the heart's workload. Wrap up well, and slowly get the big muscles of your back, buttocks and legs working so that they are making enough heat to open up the circulation before you start any hard work.

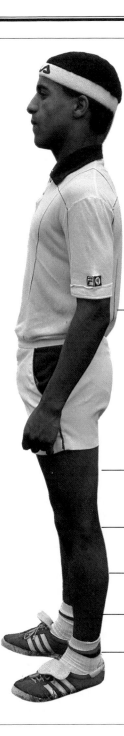

As soon as you start to train, you risk some sort of injury. Most of the problems occur in the leg muscles and tendons, and are usually the result of inadequate warming up.

Back problems are often caused by minor leg injuries which put a strain on the back muscles.

Strains and tears in the hamstrings may result from overtraining or inadequate warm-up precautions.

Minor muscle strains can put the knee under extra stress, and this may lead to injury.

Overexertion or insufficient preparation may result in strains or tears in the calf muscles.

'Shin splints' are usually caused by overtraining.

Achilles tendon injury is very common. Runners are particularly at risk, and many of the 'warm-down' exercises are designed to minimize the problem.

29

GETTING STARTED

When you set out to get fit there are two main objectives. The first is to get as fit as possible as quickly as possible, and the second – which is equally important – is to avoid injury. If you try and rush along too quickly you will certainly wind up with some injury. It may not be very serious in itself, but it is bound to slow you down.

You will be astounded at the speed with which you get fit in the early stages; because you are starting from a low baseline you are able to improve at a rate that you will never equal once you are fitter. You only have to be patient over the course of a week or two, and you will find that you can do almost twice as much as you could at the start. All this can be thrown away by pushing yourself too hard, so just ease back and enjoy it – it certainly *doesn't* have to hurt to do you good.

If you want to have a trouble-free time then there is a simple message – make haste slowly. People in their teens and twenties should be able to bring themselves up from a state of almost total inactivity to a reasonable degree of fitness within two or three months (unless they are very overweight, in which case they too will have to be very careful otherwise they will risk injury). In contrast people in their forties may take twice as long to get to the same level of fitness, and those in their sixties should expect to take twice as long again.

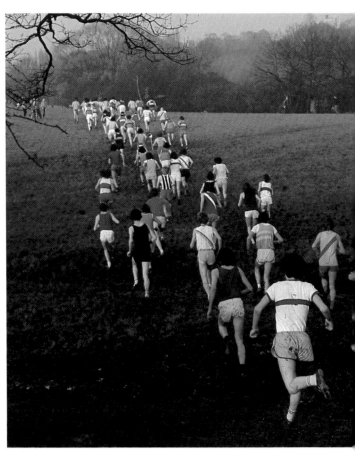

Core activities

There are many, many ways of keeping fit, but when it comes to *getting* fit it is best to concentrate on the 'big three' – walking/running, swimming and cycling. These are all highly aerobic activities that are available to almost everybody. They have the advantage that in terms of time spent, they are very efficient ways of getting fit; they will also obviously help your performance in other sports and pastimes. To these three it is reasonable to add the relatively new concept of 'aerobics',

Below: *Running is one of the most efficient ways to achieve fitness but it is important to take it easy in the early stages.*

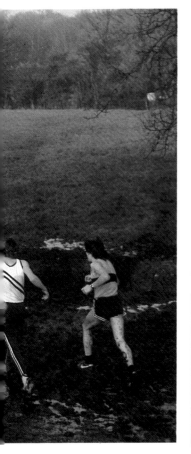

a word used to describe aerobic exercise, done to music, more or less on the spot.

Training programmes

On page 34 you will find an outline programme for getting started on running. The basic idea is to build up time and distance slowly over the course of a few weeks. The principle can be applied to any aerobic activity, and there is no need to stick rigidly to a particular scheme. The important thing to realize is that you will achieve more by building up slowly than by starting at a high level. The old adage in athletic circles is 'train don't strain' – you should not be pushing yourself all the time.

The programme on page 34 is designed for men in their mid-thirties. There is no reason why women should not proceed as fast, but it is perfectly in order to take a bit longer. If you are over the age of 40, you will definitely have to take longer, and if you are over 50 you should expect to take twice as long over each stage.

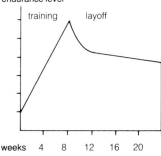

endurance level

Getting fit takes a long time, and you seem to lose that fitness distressingly quickly if you stop training. In fact things are not as bad as they seem. Although endurance falls off very quickly in the first two weeks, you retain 70 per cent of the ground you have gained for at least three months even if you do no training at all.

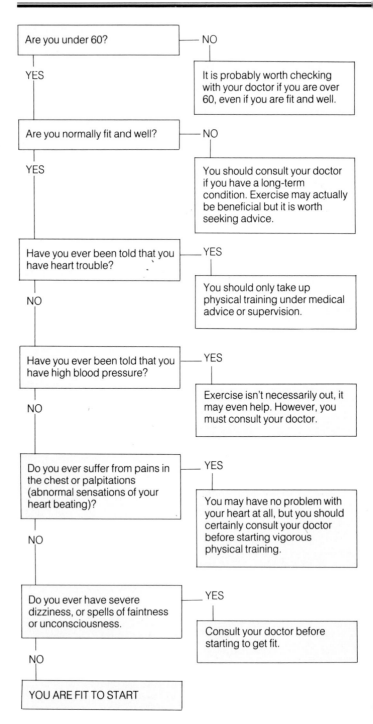

Are you under 60? — NO

YES

It is probably worth checking with your doctor if you are over 60, even if you are fit and well.

Are you normally fit and well? — NO

YES

You should consult your doctor if you have a long-term condition. Exercise may actually be beneficial but it is worth seeking advice.

Have you ever been told that you have heart trouble? — YES

NO

You should only take up physical training under medical advice or supervision.

Have you ever been told that you have high blood pressure? — YES

NO

Exercise isn't necessarily out, it may even help. However, you must consult your doctor.

Do you ever suffer from pains in the chest or palpitations (abnormal sensations of your heart beating)? — YES

NO

You may have no problem with your heart at all, but you should certainly consult your doctor before starting vigorous physical training.

Do you ever have severe dizziness, or spells of faintness or unconsciousness. — YES

NO

Consult your doctor before starting to get fit.

YOU ARE FIT TO START

OBESITY

There are problems involved in getting fit if you are overweight, and the more overweight you are, the worse the problems. The main difficulty is that your muscles, joints and bones are subjected to a much greater strain and they are therefore much more susceptible to injury.

Swimming has the great advantage that it puts much less of a strain on bones and joints; it is very much to be recommended if you are overweight. Unfortunately some people are embarrassed to go swimming if they are very fat.

If you are overweight, it will take you longer to get fit. It has been suggested that it takes over two months for very obese people to get fit enough to walk 1,5 km. However, the benefits of improved fitness are probably greater for people with a weight problem than for anyone else, so it is well worth the effort.

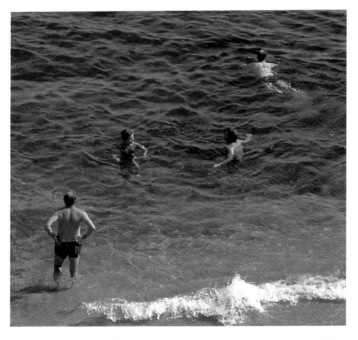

Left: *If you can follow this flow chart through without any problems, then there is no reason why you should not start out to get aerobically fit. It is important to talk to your doctor before trying to get fit if you have some long-term problem like arthritis or diabetes. He is quite likely to tell you to go ahead, but he may want to give you special advice.*

Above: *Swimming in the sun while on holiday is an excellent way to start getting fit, and it is also one of the safest if you are overweight or getting on in years. The water supports the body and minimizes the risk of straining something, and the action of swimming exercises all the major muscles of the body and improves overall flexibility.*

33

Pulse rate

It isn't necessary to take your pulse while you are training, but some people like to do so – it can be a source of considerable encouragement in the early stages. The pulse is a good indicator of overall fitness and you will find that your pulse rate slows down quite a lot over the course of a few weeks' training. The improvement in pulse rate recovery – that is to say the time it takes to get back to normal after a period of exercise – is even more striking.

The pulse rate is also a useful guide to the level of activity that does you most good. To achieve a valuable training effect you want to be working at around three-quarters of your theoretical maximum heart rate. This maximum can be found quite simply by subtracting your age from 210. For a 30-year-old, the maximum is 180, so he should be working at a rate of about 135.

There is an alternative way of assessing the best possible work level on the basis of pulse rate. Take the maximum rate and subtract your resting rate (measured over a full minute, sitting down, after five minutes' rest). Multiply this number by 0,75, add it back to your resting rate, and you have your ideal training pulse rate. Here is the formula again:

Maximum rate – resting rate = N
Ideal training rate = Resting rate + 0,75 x N

Obviously it is difficult to take your pulse while you are actually running, swimming or cycling. The thing to do is stop and take your pulse over five or ten seconds. Remember to start counting at 'nought' and not at 'one', or you will count it faster than it really is.

A running programme

This training schedule will take you from a state of very low aerobic fitness to a state where you will be able to cover 8 km at a gentle trot. The rate of progression and the timings are calculated to suit people in their mid-thirties. If you are over

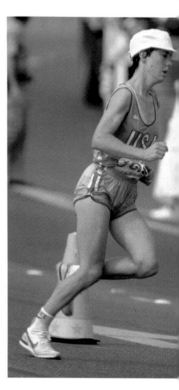

Above: *It is now thought that women have a natural aptitude for endurance events. In 1984 Joan Benoit ran the Olympic marathon in just under 2 hours 25 minutes – this would have beaten half the men who had won Olympic marathons up to then.*

45 you should do each week twice, and if you are over 60 you can expect to spend nearly a month over each stage. The target times in the last column are the least important part, and you certainly shouldn't be racing to reach a target time. There is a simple rule – if you are working so hard that you cannot talk, then slow down until you can. In the end you will get fitter quicker.

There are certain features of this training schedule which are applicable to any aerobic exercise. In this case distance has been used as the basic measure, but it is only a

A TRAINING PROGRAMME FOR RUNNING

Week	Distance	Frequency per week	Time in minutes
1	1,5 km W	5	–
2	2,5 km W 800 m W/R	3 2	– 7
3	800 m R 1,5 km W/R	2 3	6 –
4	1,5 km R 3 km W/R	3 2	11 –
5	1,5 km R 1 km R 6,5 km W	2 2 1	10,5 5 –
6	1,5 km R 3 km W/R	2 2	10 –
7	1,5 km R 2,5 km R 5 km W/R	2 2 1	9,5 16 –
8	1,5 km R 2,5 km R 5 km R	2 2 1	9 15 33
9	3 km R 5 km R 800 m W/R	2 1 1	19 32 –
10	1,5 km R 3 km R 6,5 km R	2 2 1	8,5 18 –
11	3 km R 5 km R 6,5 km R	1 2 1	17,5 30 40
12	3 km R 5 km R 8 km R	1 2 1	17,5 28,5 –

way of indicating the time that should be spent exercising.

Another thing to notice is the fact that there is no steady progression. There are easy weeks, like weeks six to nine, and there are slightly harder weeks. It is a good principle to work hard for a week and then slacken off the following week.

Those sessions marked 'W' should be carried out at a brisk walk. Those marked 'W/R' should be a mixture of walking and running, either at a gentle jog for the whole distance or walking some of the way and running the rest. Sessions marked 'R' should be carried out at a comfortable running pace.

There is no doubt that there are definite dangers associated with physical exertion. Serious injuries can occur during contact sports – they can only be prevented by suitable rules and, perhaps more important, proper umpiring and refereeing. Similarly high-speed sports such as skiing have inherant risks, and there are environmental dangers involved in many of the outdoor sports such as sailing and mountaineering. Swimming, although remarkably free from minor injury problems, carries the risk of drowning, but once again this can be reduced by taking simple precautions.

Most people take such risks for granted, and even enjoy the sense of adventure they inspire, but exercise can lead to other problems which are at best irritating, and at worst can cause permanent, even fatal damage to the body. Luckily these problems are easy to avoid if you take care.

Minor problems
These involve injury to muscles, joints, tendons, or ligaments. Often these injuries result from over-training and pushing yourself too hard. This applies to running injuries in particular. It is vital to ease

Right: *Problems at work can create problems in training. Tension increases the risk of injury, so ease off if you are under stress.* Below right: *Extremes of heat or cold make injury more likely. Cut back on training in hot or cold weather until you acclimatize.*

STOP if...
- you get a pain in the chest
- you start to feel sick
- your breathing becomes much more laboured and difficult than usual
- you start to feel as though you are overheating, and start getting very hot
- you feel unwell in any other way

It is vital to watch out for signs of problems in the brain or nervous system so:

STOP if...
- you feel dizzy or you start to become confused
- you develop a severe headache whilst exercising
- you notice any difficulty moving part of your body, or the sensation becomes abnormal
- you become uncoordinated and can't walk or run in a straight line

WATCH OUT if...
you have a cold or similar minor illness. Keep any training to a minimum. NEVER go in for any sort of competition or race with a cold or 'flu – however long you may have been in training for it.

ALWAYS...
make sure you have done enough training for any race or competition you enter. If you haven't, then just withdraw – it isn't worth risking your health.

NEVER...
make a sudden increase in the amount of work you do even if you have some unexpected time off – it is a sure way to pick up an injury of some description.

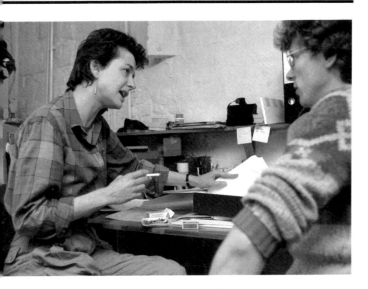

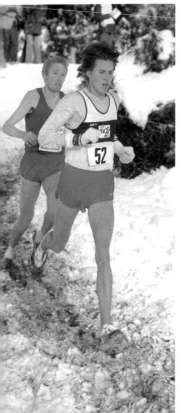

off if you injure yourself – or you may suffer months of discomfort and relative inactivity.

Major problems

Serious damage involving collapse of the heart and circulation and other major difficulties are to a large extent preventable. The biggest risk is to people who are known to have some sort of heart problem, so before starting a fitness programme go through the chart on page 32 very carefully. When you are training it is most important to respond sensibly to the messages from your body, and the danger signals and recommendations are listed on the opposite page.

The risk of sudden death whilst exercising has been widely discussed in the press. The most informative study so far has come from Auckland, New Zealand where a population of 5000 was studied. It turned out that only a tiny fraction of those who died suddenly – 3½ per cent in fact – were regular exercisers. This represented five people, all of whom were known to have heart disease.

CORE ACTIVITIES

Digging potatoes in the garden, or running up a flight of stairs with a pile of washing, does not fit in with the conventional image of physical exercise. Nevertheless, ordinary everyday activities can contribute a lot to aerobic training, and the way you organize your daily routine can have a significant effect on your state of fitness.

Furthermore, most people find that a certain amount of aerobic training makes them a lot fitter than they were before, and it then becomes easier to adopt a more active approach to the business of everyday life. If you are rather unfit it is impossible to summon the enthusiasm to climb two flights of stairs when there is a perfectly good lift to take you, but once you are fit it ceases to be a problem. Stair-climbing is in fact a very good form of aerobic exercise, which involves about the same level of exertion as running at a relaxed pace.

Activities such as gardening, and

A group of sedentary middle aged office workers agreed to stop using the lift for a trial period. During the study they climbed an average of 25 flights of stairs each day. With no other exercise this led to an increase in endurance fitness of 15 per cent after ten weeks.

even ordinary housework, are also energetic, and therefore they are quite beneficial in terms of aerobic training. The more you exercise your body and burn up energy, the fitter you get – indeed, you are actually burning about 50 per cent more energy when you are standing up than when you are sitting down.

Similarly you can add a lot to your level of fitness by making sure you walk as much as possible, and resisting the impulse to take a car or some sort of public transport. The bicycle, of course, provides another excellent means of getting – and staying – aerobically fit, and regular cycling can be fitted easily into your everyday life.

Below: *You don't have to be wearing a tracksuit to be keeping fit. Gardening can be a very good way to get exercise.*

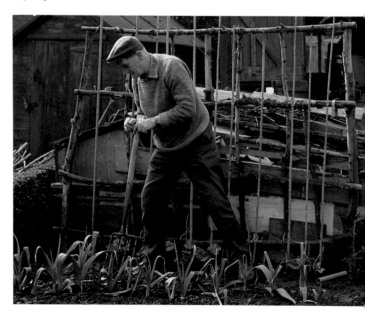

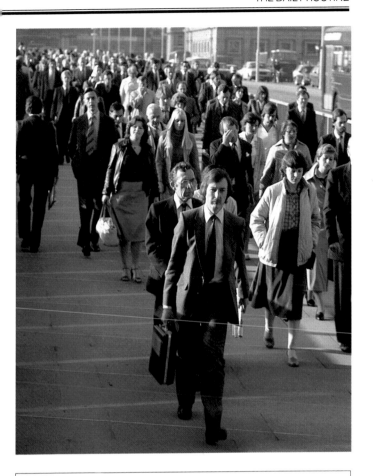

Mr Potter and Mr Slump live in the same suburb, and they both work in the same office in town. Mr Potter takes the train to and from work; this involves a walk of a kilometre from home to the station, and half a kilometre at the other end – he therefore walks 3 km a day to and from the office. Mr Slump drives to work.

Mr Potter works on the third floor of the office block while Mr Slump works on the fifth floor. They collaborate closely, so they have to visit each other's offices two or three times a day. Mr Potter goes up and down the stairs, while Mr Slump takes the lift.

As a result of these minor differences in a lifestyle that is otherwise almost identical, Mr Potter's daily energy output is enough to have a significant training effect, whereas Mr Slump's has very little. During the course of his ordinary working day Mr Potter burns off an extra 840 kJ, so during one working week he burns an extra 4200 kJ. In order to catch up with this level of energy expenditure, Mr Slump would have to jog for about two hours, and even if he did, it is far from certain that the overall effect of this form of training, once or twice a week, would be as beneficial as the regular activities of Mr Potter.

For many people, running provides an ideal form of exercise. It is certainly one of the things that the human body is designed to do well: humans are not as fast as many other animals, but there are few species which can keep going for as long or as far. It is convenient and efficient, and there are many unexpected advantages as you become a reasonably fit runner. For example it is a very healthy way of relaxing after a day's work, and it provides an unbeatable way of seeing new places. You can stop and explore whenever you like, having no car to park or bike to lock, then carry on where you left off.

Running – or jogging as some prefer to call it – needs only the minimum of equipment. The only important requirement is a good pair of training shoes, but there is no need to buy the most expensive. Apart from this you can run in almost any type of clothing, although loose tracksuits in colder weather or shorts and singlets in warmer weather are the ideal.

There is a simple starting programme on page 35 which provides a guide to starting out on running as regular exercise. The essence of training for simple fitness and enjoyment is to go for distance and not to worry about speed – that will come later if you get keen.

Aerobics

Aerobics is a new word, but not a new idea. The old concept of calisthenics or 'physical jerks' was essentially the same. Both involve various exercises which are not too energetic, but repeated many times they result in an excellent form of aerobic training which improves flexibility as well as aerobic fitness. In aerobics the calisthenics are performed to a rhythmic pulse of disco music and strung together in what amounts to a modern dance form – so making the exercise more enjoyable and encouraging extra effort.

> A study of 'aerobics' compared to running was carried out among 46 previously untrained women. It was found that four sessions per week for seven weeks produced the same improvement of capacity in the aerobics group as it did in the runners.

You can do aerobics on your own, for there are usually regular aerobics sessions broadcast on television; alternatively you can buy records and tapes complete with instructions and music. However, most people do their aerobics in classes, in the gyms and 'Aerobics Studios' which are available – at least in towns and cities. It isn't necessarily cheap, but it is a sociable and effective way of increasing fitness which many people enjoy. Aerobics classes are just as good for men as for women, but it is mostly women who take advantage of them.

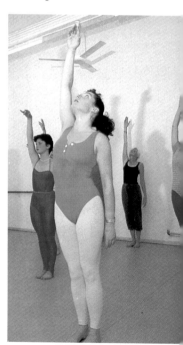

RUNNING TIPS

● Keep yourself warm – particularly the upper part of your body. Some people feel comfortable running in shorts even in the coldest weather, but in such conditions it is important to wear plenty of layers above the waist. Gloves are essential for comfortable running in cold weather.

● Don't try to run on your toes; let your heel strike the ground first. Other than this, don't think too much about the way you are running – let your style develop naturally.

● Try to vary the surfaces you run over, keeping tarmac to a minimum when you are in the early stages.

● Try to vary the terrain, alternating between flat ground, gentle undulations and steep hills as often as possible (it doesn't matter at all if you walk up the steep parts). This will bring all the various muscle groups into play.

● Running does little for your flexibility, so remember the warm-up and warm-down exercises which are designed to keep your muscles on the stretch.

● It is well worth running with a friend or friends from time to time – it makes a change and often speeds up your progress to fitness.

Left: *Attending an aerobics class is a very effective form of training. The exercises improve flexibility and shape as well as aerobic capacity, and the music encourages you to stick at it.*

Below: *A well-designed pair of training shoes is the only equipment you need for running. They will not only be more comfortable, they will reduce the frequency of minor injuries.*

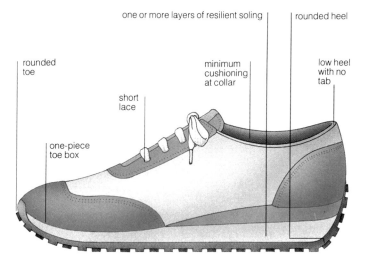

one or more layers of resilient soling

rounded heel

rounded toe

minimum cushioning at collar

low heel with no tab

short lace

one-piece toe box

As a form of aerobic training, swimming has almost everything. Indeed, it is such a good way of getting fit, it is advisable to try and include a weekly swimming session as part of every fitness programme. Swimming has three main advantages over almost any other sort of training:

● Swimming improves all the major elements of fitness: aerobic fitness, muscle strength *and* flexibility.

● Unlike many other forms of training, swimming exercises all your muscles, especially your arms, and this adds to your overall energy output.

● Despite the high energy levels involved the risk of injury is very low, because the water cushions you from the effects of gravity. Because of this, swimming is especially valuable if you are overweight, or if you are pregnant.

The level of exertion when you swim is quite high – provided that you don't simply lie around floating in the pool, so it is an efficient form of aerobic training.

Furthermore you don't need anything more than a swimming costume, although naturally you have to have access to a pool.

Swimming does have some disadvantages, however, and the obvious one is that you may not have learned to swim. It is never too late to learn, though, and many people have started swimming in their sixties or seventies. Swimming also seems to be one of the areas where individuals differ very greatly – some people may be very athletic in other areas, but they never learn to swim very fast. You may see one swimmer streaking through the water, while another is working hard but going at only half the speed. It is important to realize that it is the overall energy output which matters, and that the training effect may well be the same in both individuals.

Below: *Swimming ability is essential for water sports, so the sooner children learn to swim, the better.*

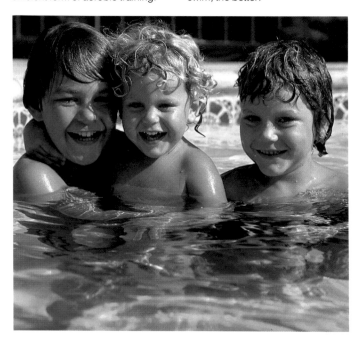

Many people find that a swim three or four times every week is all that they need to keep fit. Others find it difficult to keep up their enthusiasm, since swimming up and down the same pool is less interesting than running through varied surroundings. Variation of style and stroke may help in this respect.

Style and strokes

The four strokes used in competitive swimming are the front crawl (freestyle), back crawl (backstroke), breast stroke and butterfly. Many swimmers never manage to master more than a few strokes of butterfly, and some people cannot keep up a sustained front crawl for more than a minute or so, although practice helps.

You will achieve a perfectly adequate level of aerobic training if you stick to the breast stroke.

Below: *The aerobic value of swimming depends on how hard you work. This butterfly swimmer is working very hard indeed.*

To compare the performance of a runner and a swimmer simply multiply by four – for freestyle swimming at any rate. A top-class swimmer will cover half a kilometre in the same time that a runner takes to cover 2 km.

The advantage of switching from stroke to stroke, apart from keeping up your interest, is that you use different groups of muscles, and put joints through different sets of movements. This all helps to increase the flexibility of your body. Another point to bear in mind is that butterfly and front crawl involve a great deal of energy expenditure, and it is quite difficult to allow yourself to slacken off in either of these strokes. On the other hand an experienced breast stroke swimmer can let himself slow down to the extent that he is barely using more energy than walking. This ability is useful when you start training.

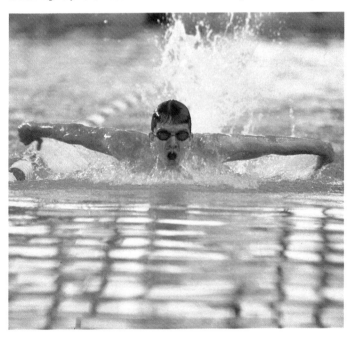

The bicycle is an exceptional invention. There is no more effective way of harnessing human muscle power – a man on a bicycle is the most efficient system in the animal and mechanical worlds in terms of the amount of energy used to cover a given distance on the flat. The aircraft *Gossamer Albatross,* which made a successful crossing of the English Channel in 1979, was propelled by manpower alone using basic bicycle design to harness the muscular energy of its pilot, Bryan Allen.

In some respects the bicycle's very efficiency creates problems as a means of getting fit. It is so efficient that, under some circumstances, it is possible to keep moving at reasonable speeds while using no more muscular effort than that involved in going for a gentle stroll. When you are riding a bicycle on a flat surface, the work you are doing is acting on three things: any friction in the machinery, the rolling resistance of the tyres against the road surface, and wind resistance. On a good modern bicycle the first two

factors should be minimal, so you are basically working against wind resistance. This of course depends very much on how fast you are going, and in fact you only have to slow down by a few miles per hour to halve the level of wind resistance and therefore halve the amount of work that you hare having to do.

The importance of wind resistance is very apparent in a big cycle race like the Tour de France, where the tactics depend upon slipstreaming the opposition as much as possible – that is, cycling just behind one's opponent so that he does all the work of forcing a passage through the air. Cyclists can get up to very

Right: *If you merely coast on the flat you don't have to put much effort into cycling, but a road-racing cyclist will use a great deal of energy and achieve a very high level of aerobic fitness.* Below: *The bicycle is a great liberator – touring by bike is probably the best way of getting to know the countryside. It gets you fit, too.*

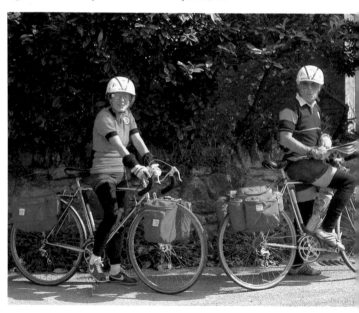

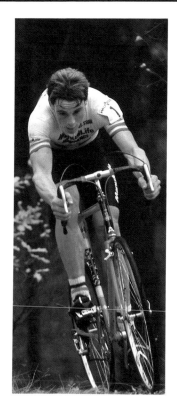

bad; rolling resistance is kept to a minimum by inflating the tyres really hard. As you improve you may well want to get a lightweight bike; the weight of the bike doesn't matter on the flat, but it makes a tremendous difference on any sort of hill. (This is one reason why racing bikes are so light; a light bike is also easier to accelerate which is important in competition.)

Most bikes have gears, and these certainly help on hills. If you have a ten-speed bike, try and increase your pedalling speed as much as possible to begin with. Don't push too hard on a hill, but drop a gear and let your legs go around faster. Apart from anything else, it puts less of a strain on the transmission of the bike.

Keep fit machines

Many different types of keep fit machine are sold for people to use at home. The commonest are exercise bikes and rowing machines. Both machines are certainly very effective at keeping you aerobically fit – assuming you are disciplined enough to keep to a daily session while you are getting fit, and a session three or four times a week to keep fit. In reality it is very hard to keep up this sort of discipline, because the process of pedalling away on an exercise bike, or pulling away on a rowing machine, soon loses its appeal.

This is much less of a problem with the other core activities. Nevertheless, if the idea appeals to you and you can afford the price, using exercise machines may be an effective way to get you started on a successful fitness programme.

high speeds by following an appropriate motor vehicle, although this is obviously very dangerous on ordinary roads.

Once you start having to climb hills you need to do a lot of work against gravity and this increases the aerobic training effect. Wherever possible it is a good idea to include hills in any programme of cycling training. Apart from the extra work involved, it also brings different muscles into play, particularly if you use the 'honking' (standing up on the pedals) approach.

You can start to cycle on any bike that fits you. The most important dimension is the distance from saddle to pedal which should be slightly more than the length of your inside leg. If the bike is in reasonably good mechanical order, and well lubricated, the friction of the machinery will not be too

Bicycles are very efficient. 4 200 kJ will take the average runner about 13 km in 100 minutes, whereas the same amount of energy will take the average cyclist 40 km in the same time.

SHAPE AND STRENGTH

Shape

If you concentrate on improving your aerobic fitness you will inevitably increase your muscle strength; as a result of this you may well find that your figure becomes more pleasing. You may want to try and put a little extra effort into improving your figure, however, and there is no doubt that training all the various muscle groups of your body will help your appearance as well as your strength and aerobic capacity.

On the next page there are a number of exercises which are particularly effective for improving your figure. Of themselves they are not necessarily a recipe for overall fitness, but when added to some aerobic training they certainly help to shape you up a bit further. The advantage of doing the various 'aerobics' routines which are readily accessible these days is that most of the exercises involved are designed to help body shape, as well as ensure that the overall level of muscular activity is high enough to have a very significant training effect.

Strength

Men are usually less interested in shape for its own sake, and more interested in muscle strength. This is a rather more problematic area for it involves exercises that have little aerobic training value considering the energy used.

There is a tendency for people to muddle the two ideas of aerobic fitness and muscle strength. This is entirely understandable, since there is obviously some overlap between the two, and it is impossible to keep up a high level of energy expenditure doing body building exercises without having some sort of training effect on the heart and lungs. Nevertheless there is no evidence to suggest that increasing your total bulk of muscle makes you any healthier. It is important to have clear objectives – if you want to become bigger and stronger for some

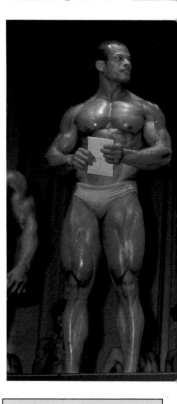

Contrary to some popular beliefs, top-class body builders are very strong indeed, but there is some doubt about other aspects of their fitness. In one study they were found to be no more flexible than average, and the aerobic fitness of those who did no aerobic training was no greater than the average for their age.

reason then it is reasonable to set out on a strength training programme, bearing in mind that some types of training are far from safe (see page 50). On the other hand if you principally want to feel good, stay as healthy as possible and maybe even do something to increase your life-span, then you should go for one of the simpler forms of aerobic training.

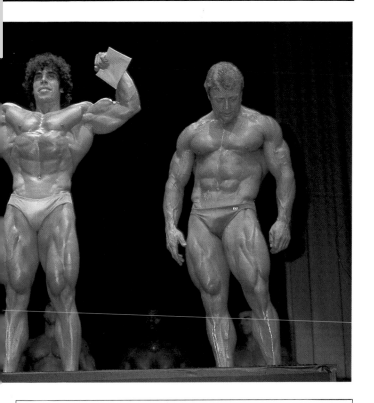

BACK STRENGTH

Back trouble is very common indeed, and the fitter members of society seem no less likely to suffer from back problems than the less fit. An increased level of physical acitivity increases the risk of all injuries including injury to the back, so in some respects fit people may be more at risk. Obviously it would be a good thing if you could reduce the probability of trouble in the future.

The muscles of the back are functionally different from most of the other muscles of the body. They run up the side of the spine, and they are responsible for holding it rigid while movement takes place in the rest of the body. Because of the way they work, they are in action most of the time – even when you are sitting down. Unlike other muscles, therefore, they are unlikely to suffer from underuse. For this reason there is no need to do special exercises to strengthen them – if you try to do this you may very well do more harm than good.

However, the muscles alongside the spine are not the only ones concerned with the shape and posture of the back – the muscles of the abdominal wall are also very important in distributing the effort involved in maintaining posture. Unlike the back muscles these can get underused and weak, and this puts more strain on the back itself which may give trouble as a result. It is well worth strengthening these muscles, and the sit-up exercises on page 25 are ideal.

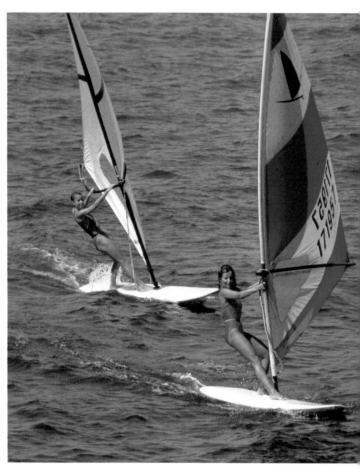

Above: *Windsurfing works all your muscles and provides you with lots of aerobic exercise – it's fun and it keeps you in shape.*

Below: *Chair Exercise. To help get your stomach muscles in trim, simply sit on a chair and draw your legs up towards your chest.*

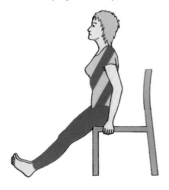 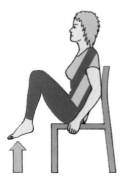

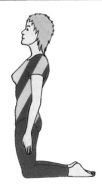
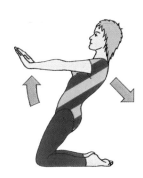

Above: *Zeds. This exercise is great for firming up the thighs. Kneel up straight, then lean back while raising your arms. Hold for* a count of two, then straighten up again. Make sure you keep your back hollowed, and knees, hips and shoulders in a straight line.

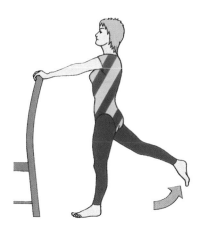
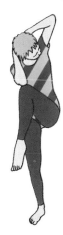

Above: *Backwards Lifts. Lift one leg backwards and outwards at 45° while steadying yourself. Relax, repeat 20 times; now change legs.*

Above: *Knee Curls. Clasp your hands behind your head, and try to touch your elbow with the opposite knee. Then change sides.*

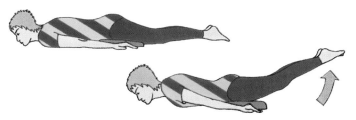

Above: *Reverse Curls. Lie face down with your hands beside you. Point your toes and raise your legs as high as you can.*

Hold for a count of five, then lower gently and repeat. Like the Backwards Lifts, this helps to trim the buttocks.

If you do go in for regular aerobic training you will probably feel that your legs are in no great need of strength training – all aerobic training involves the legs, after all. You may well wish to develop your upper body strength, however. There is no need to use fancy equipment to do this, since the safest approach to strength training is to use your own body weight to put extra load on the muscles you are interested in.

All training depends on making the muscles work. The idea behind aerobic training is to make as many muscles as possible work at the same time. All the muscles are working together and no particular group has a very heavy load. Each movement is repeated many times at these moderate loads, improving the stamina of the muscles involved, and developing the slow twitch fibres.

In contrast the idea behind strength training is to take a smaller number of muscles and put them through a much higher level of work at higher loads. There may

> *Sedentary individuals can expect to lose 15 per cent of their muscle strength between the ages of 45 and 60. If they exercise and keep reasonably fit, though, their loss of strength will be minimal.*

be very little load on other parts of the body. Furthermore the action is not repeated so often. This improves muscle power, developing the fast twitch fibres.

This approach is taken to extremes in a technique of muscle strengthening called isometric exercise. Here the idea is to make a muscle work against its maximum load for as long as possible with no period of relaxation. A typical exercise might involve putting your two hands palm to palm in front of your chest, and then pressing as hard as you can for as long as you can. There are various devices available which enable you to put all your muscle groups through isometric exercise – the best known

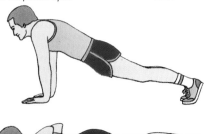

Right: *Half Press-Ups. Press-ups are excellent for strengthening arms (particularly the triceps) and shoulders. However, rather than starting with full press-ups, first try just raising the top half of your body from your knees upwards. When you can do 20, move on to full press-ups.*

Left: *Full Press-Ups. Place your palms flat on the ground under your shoulders. Straighten your arms and as you raise your body, try to keep ankles, knees, hips and shoulders in a straight line. Lower yourself gently until your chest just touches the ground, and repeat. Try to do it 20 times.*

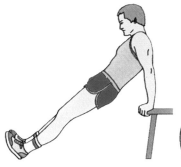

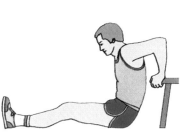

Above: *Chair dips. These help to strengthen the back of the arms and the shoulders. Gripping the front edge of a chair, stretch your legs out while resting on your heels, then raise yourself*

up with your arms straight. Now let yourself down as though you are going to sit on the ground. As you touch the ground push yourself back up again into the starting position.

is the Bullworker. The problem with isometric exercise is that it does nothing for the circulation. It may even cause problems, since isometric activity in the arms puts the blood pressure up.

Most people think of weight training as soon as mucle strength is mentioned, but such apparatus is quite unnecessary. Indeed, training with free weights can be dangerous – if you were to buy a set from a mail order catalogue and start off unsupervised you would be unlikely to escape some sort of muscle injury. Free weights have in any case become redundant with the availability of 'multigym' apparatus, where the weights are operated through rope and pulley devices which make them much more controllable.

In the last few years there has been a development in the use of 'isokinetic' training. This involves carefully designed machines which are able to provide a constant load on the muscle throughout its range of movement. The load can be varied, and therefore the extent to which it produces power or stamina effects. There is also very little risk of injury. The only disadvantage is that the machines are expensive, and a different machine is needed for each muscle group.

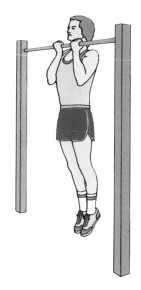

Above: *Pull-ups. These are the best way of strengthening your forearms and your biceps. You will need a bar at just over head height – you can fit one in a doorway. Simply pull yourself up so your chin is over the bar, and try not to cheat by jumping off the ground. Grasp the bar with the backs of your hands towards you for the first few pull-ups, then switch so the palms are facing you.*

FITNESS THROUGHOUT LIFE

In ideal circumstances, the problem during pregnancy should be one of *keeping* fit rather than *getting* fit. Pregnancy is not the ideal time to start out on a vigorous exercise programme in order to get fit, and it is much better to postpone any major effort to achieve fitness until later. That said, it is certainly worth trying to improve on things a little by some sort of aerobic exercise.

If you do not usually engage in any sporting activity then the best things for you are probably walking and swimming. Swimming is very good exercise for anyone who is pregnant, since it puts very little strain on the bones and joints. It has another important advantage for mothers who already have children, since it is ideal for small children who want to join in.

After delivery

The first few weeks after delivery are obviously very busy, and your thoughts are very much centred around the new baby, but eventually you will want to start getting your figure back.

You should not start on this too early, and it is perhaps best to leave it until after your first postnatal visit to the clinic. Once you have had a check-up, you can begin to work on the muscles of your abdomen. The best exercises to get your abdomen in trim are the situps shown on pages 25 and 48. Good firm abdominal muscles will also help your back, which carries as much strain with a new baby as it does during pregnancy.

During pregnancy it is very important not to exercise at an excessive level. There is a simple rule of thumb: whatever form of exercise you are engaged in, it will be doing you good without the risk of harm provided that you still have enough breath left to carry out a normal conversation.

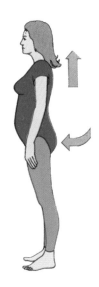

Above: *This simple exercise will protect your back. Tuck your bottom in and stretch up with your back, several times a day.*

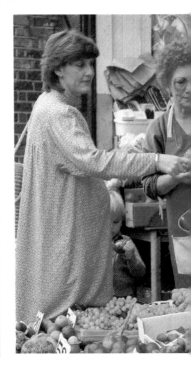

Q If you exercise too much during pregnancy, is there any likelihood of harming the baby?

A No. Obviously you have to be sensible, and avoid really heavy exertion in pregnancy – you shouldn't be training for a marathon. Later on in pregnancy you yourself are more at risk than the baby, since your increased size and weight can cause problems.

Q Will exercise help during the process of birth?

A Many people believe that giving birth is easier if you are fit, but there is no clearcut scientific evidence that will back this up. Pregnancy is like any other time of life in this respect – you will probably feel better if you are physically fit.

Q Are there any parts of the body which are put under special strain by pregnancy?

A The pelvis and its muscles are obviously under stress; the abdominal wall is also stretched, and it is a good idea to try and strengthen it again after delivery. Another area which bears a lot of strain is the back. Exercises such as the one on this page can help, but perhaps more important is to avoid wearing high heels which disrupt your posture and put your back under even more strain. Your legs and ankles also tend to swell during pregnancy, so try to avoid standing for long periods.

Below left: *You need stamina during pregnancy to get through all the jobs you have to do, so being fit is a great asset.*

Below: *Swimming is the safest and most effective form of exercise when you are pregnant – toddlers can join in too.*

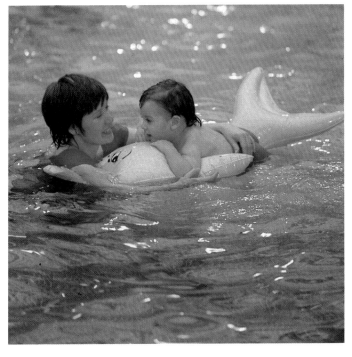

In the womb

Babies start to exercise their muscles long before they are born. Every expectant mother knows that the baby's kicks are a good sign – they help to develop the muscles of the arms and the legs. Now that we are able to look at babies in the womb using sophisticated scanning techniques, it is clear that towards the end of pregnancy they are very active indeed. Not only do they kick out with their arms and legs, but they also go through the movements of breathing and crying – using muscles that need exercise to develop properly.

Babies

Babies and small children need no encouragement to take all the exercise that is good for them – all they really need is the opportunity. Anyone who has ever had to change a nappy knows that babies love to kick their legs around as soon as they are free from restrictions. This kicking is good for the developing muscles, and it obviously gives huge enjoyment. As they grow older they remain very active and most parents wonder where all that energy comes from. Of course some babies are more active than others, and there is a lot of variation in the ages when individual children pass the major milestones, such as learning to walk.

The arrival of a small baby obviously makes a lot of difference to the leisure activity of the parents, but there is no need to give up taking useful outdoor exercise together. There are many excellent backpacks and slings available to carry your baby or

Right: *Walking is one of the best ways to keep fit, and a baby or toddler taken along in a sling is very little hindrance.*
Below: *Taking the whole family for a cycle ride provides useful exercise, and encourages small children to join in when they can.*

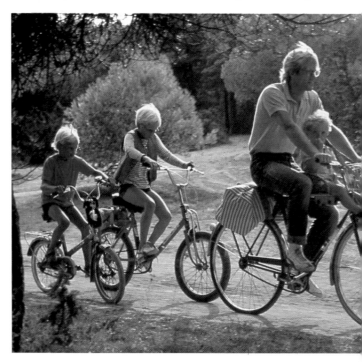

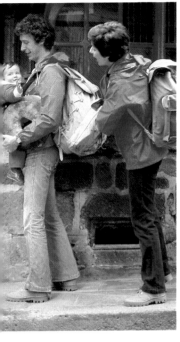

even a good-sized toddler. In fact some couples don't discover the fun of rambling until the arrival of their first baby. Similarly you can carry babies and small children on a bicycle, although it is sensible to restrict such activities to the very quietest roads, and use a well-designed child's seat.

Toddlers

Most parents find the toddler stage the most exciting and attractive period of their child's development. There is no real necessity to provide more than the opportunity for most of them to get all the exercise they need, but it is quite a good idea to start introducing some of the skills that make sports of all sorts enjoyable. It is never too early to take babies or toddlers swimming, and get them used to the water. You can also introduce a ball and let them play with it.

A word of warning, though: very small children learn almost exclusively by play. Overambitious parents who push too hard to get their child swimming or kicking a football are as likely to put him off as to produce a star of the future. Toddlers like to do things with their parents, and if they enjoy themselves all is well and they learn all they need. Push them too hard and you will only slow things down.

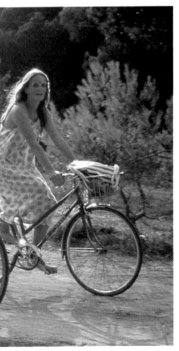

In a Canadian survey of fitness it was found that people between the ages of 2 and 17 spent a total of more than 20 hours a week in front of the television. The older schoolchildren were found to be sitting at a desk for 90 per cent of their school week. (Another survey showed that some of these children had watched an amazing 8,000 hours of food commercials on television, over three-quarters of which were selling food of low nutritional value.)

Encouraging a positive attitude

As a general rule, children don't need to work at keeping fit in the way that adults do. Left alone, young children keep up a high level of physical activity – quite high enough to keep them fit. However, there is a tendency for children to be less fit than they used to be. They spend more time sitting down in front of television sets, so they have less time to play games.

The first priority for young children is to build up a positive attitude to exercise and physical exertion. Luckily this is as natural as breathing to most children, and all you have to do is encourage it. The more that parents take part in games of all sorts, whether they are simple running games or games with a ball, the more the children will want to play similar active games themselves.

Building up skills

Once children start at school, they begin a period of formal physical education, although they spend less time on it than on other types of school work. The attitude of parents is vital to the way that they progress. If you spend time reading with a child, you encourage him to see that the school and family share the same aims. In the same way you can encourage participation in school sport by spending a little time kicking a football, organising a few races between different members of the family or doing a little catching practice. The object is to prevent the child getting the idea that sport is something childish, that adults simple don't do.

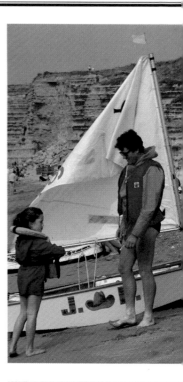

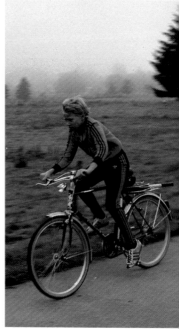

Top right: *Children are quick to pick up any new activity, and teaching them is very satisfying.*
Right: *Cycling is an essential skill – it keeps children active and gives them independence.*

There is a basic minimum of physical skills that a child
needs so that he or she will be equipped to enjoy a physically
active lifestyle as a teenager or an adult.

Swimming
Everybody should be able to swim. If you can't swim then most water
sports are impossible. The ideal is to teach your children to swim
yourself, although most schools now teach swimming. Either way
you should have your child swimming well by the age of ten.

Cycling
Everybody should also be able to ride a bicycle, and most children
will want to be taught before they go to school. This is something
you will almost certainly have to do yourself. Most children will have
learnt to pedal on a tricycle or a two-wheeler with stabilisers. When
the time comes to progress, a few hours' practice is usually enough.

Obviously children fall off as they are learning, and it will destroy
their confidence if they hurt themselves too much. You can't get
over this by practising on grass, since it is a good deal harder to
cycle on than a smooth surface. The trick is to get the child to put
on good thick long trousers and gloves, so the tumbles don't hurt.

Ball skills
There are few areas where people differ so strikingly as in their
skill at various ball games, but it is good idea to work on these skills
even if they are not your child's strongest point. For young
children, simple kicking and catching games are best.

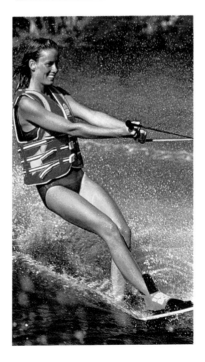

Left: *Some sports such as
water-skiing are learnt much
more quickly in childhood.*

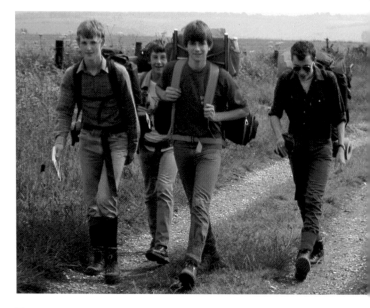

Above: *A sport does not have to be competitive to provide valuable exercise.*

Most people are at their most physically active in their teens and in their twenties. If there is a sport that they play, these are the years when they play it most regularly. Most competitive sportsmen and women – whether professional or amateur – fall into this age group, and it is this element of competition which is the real spur to physical fitness. Competitiveness is therefore well worth encouraging, but there are a number of problems with it.

The first problem is that the edge inevitably wears off your competitive instinct during your twenties and thirties. As a result of this, and of the other pressures that build up in your life, you are likely to give up sport between the ages of 30 and 40. This, of course, is the time when it is most important to be taking regular exercise, for it is very much more difficult to get fit again after 35 than it was before.

An even bigger problem is the fact that competition can be discouraging as well as encouraging, because if you are not particularly good at sport then you obviously don't want to get beaten all the time. If fitness relies on the competitive instinct, we are left with the situation which has existed for many years – naturally good sportsmen remain fit after they leave school and the rest of us become physically inactive and very unfit.

The answer is to consider a much broader range of sports, so that all teenagers, regardless of conventional sporting ability, can become interested in some sort of physical activity. It is very important to identify teenagers who are not particularly interested in, for example, football or netball. Rather than trying to make them stay, bored and shivering, on the football field or the netball court, it is better to encourage them to look at something else. If they can find something that depends neither on direct competition, nor on ball-skills, their interest in physical activity may be re-awakened. Water sports, and outdoor activities such as hill walking, climbing or orienteering

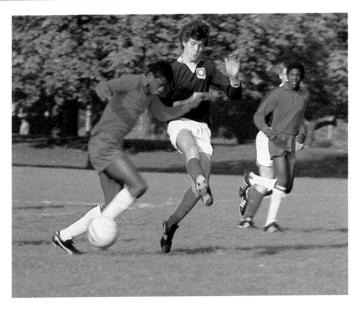

Above: *Competitive sports appeal to many teenagers and provide a good incentive to get fit.*

often appeal strongly to people who are not attracted to ball-games and team sports.

Grooming a champion?

Many parents nurse a dream that their child is a potential champion, and they may even worry that they are failing to provide adequate opportunities. Such parents should realize that for every ten, or even hundred young people who have been pushed hard to train during their teenage years, only one or two turn out to be national or world class sportsmen. It isn't necessarily the best upbringing for the others.

There is a lot to be said for allowing real sporting talent to emerge naturally. A country like East Germany produces sports champions by looking at the potential sporting skills of almost all its youth. In contrast a country like Britain, which is still rooted in 'the amateur tradition' produces many fewer champions – but those that do emerge are of truly inspirational quality. Steve Ovett and Sebastian Coe are good examples. If you look at Bjorn Borg – one of the most exciting champions of recent years – you see someone raised in a country with no great tradition of his chosen sport. These sportsmen have true star quality, whereas the products of the mechanistic selection systems used in countries like East Germany have much less charisma, despite their sporting prowess. In view of this it is probably best to settle for encouraging a reasonable degree of physical activity in the whole community, and let the champions emerge by themselves.

The risk of developing heart disease can be identified early in life. One study showed that 40 per cent of American children had some identifiable risk such as high cholesterol levels, obesity or poor measured aerobic capacity. 10 per cent of these children were at risk because of regular cigarette smoking.

Unless you are in the habit of taking regular exercise, or unless your daily work involves a lot of physical effort, you will wake up some time between the ages of 35 and 50 to the realization that you have become so unfit that even everyday activities leave you exhausted. You may find for example that the effort of walking up a couple of flights of stairs leaves you panting at the top. Or you may discover that the simple effort of bending down to tie up a shoelace leaves you embarrased by your shortness of breath.

People often think that this problem is confined to men, but it is not so. It is true that many of the activities which make up a high proportion of a housewife's day have a considerable training effect, and this can certainly delay any decline in physical fitness, but later on in life the problem of inactivity and subsequent deterioration is if anything worse in women than in men.

It doesn't take very long for your level of fitness to decline. Even if you were very fit and athletic in your twenties, if you stop all training it will only be ten years or so before you find yourself just as unfit as someone who has done no exercise since leaving school.

It must be emphasized that there is more to your overall well-being than the amount of exercise you take. You will find yourself in trouble all the sooner if you are a smoker – there is little doubt that if you wished to find the single most effective way of sabotaging your own health then smoking is the vice to choose. Not only does it have a serious effect on the heart and blood vessels, making a major contribution to the risk of heart attacks and strokes, it also has a very striking effect on the lungs. Cigarette smoke tends to destroy the elastic omponents within the lungs so that they are less pliable for the muscles of respiration to work on. In a nutshell this means the lungs are aged well before

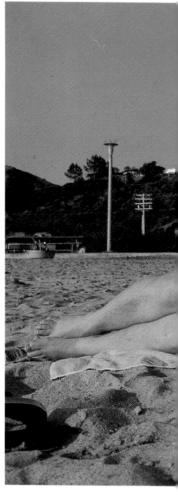

their time – a heavy smoker of 35 has the lungs of a non-smoking 60-year-old.

Being overweight will also bring forward the moment when you suddenly realize that your body is not what it was. This effect is most marked in people who are very overweight – that is, more than 20 per cent over their ideal body weight.

The solution
All this may make you feel discouraged, but you don't have to worry. The message is a

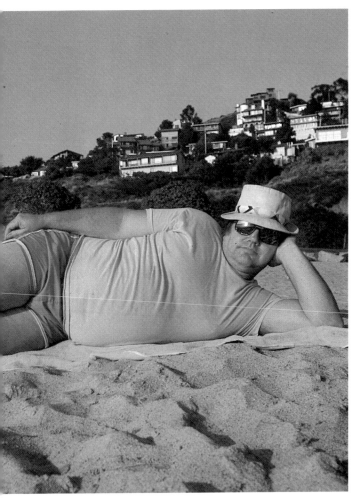

simple one – it is never too late to get fit. What is more, a 50-year-old is more likely to succeed in getting fit than a 30-year-old. There is no doubt that the 50-year-old will have to proceed more slowly, and it will certainly take him more than twice as long to reach the same level of fitness even if the two people are starting from the same level. Experience shows, however, that 50-year-olds have fewer distractions and perhaps greater tenacity, so they may be more likely to reach their goal in the end.

Above: *A little overindulgence, a sedentary lifestyle, and you too can have a body like this!*

Smoking is probably the most serious risk to health in the middle years. All forms of aerobic exercise help people to give up – in a study of runners who smoked when they started running, three-quarters of them had given up, the men being more successful at stopping than the women.

If you think of all the elderly people that you know, you will realize that some seem very hale and hearty and almost as active in their eighties as they were in their sixties, but there are other, less fortunate people who slow down and become very restricted in their activities when they are only just over 70.

Of course there are many possible reasons for elderly people slowing down and doing less – unavoidable illness is often to blame – but there is a common belief that fit, active people in their eighties are very lucky to be healthy enough to keep going. In fact, luck probably has very little to do with it – people who remain fit and healthy in their later years almost certainly do so *because* they keep up a high level of physical activity.

If you are starting on a fitness programme in your later years the important thing is to proceed very slowly. The same principles apply in this age-group as they do earlier on – the way to avoid injury is to build up slowly (see page 30). Few people in their seventies will want to take up running, although there is no particular reason why they shouldn't, but walking, cycling and especially swimming are as effective in the later years as they are earlier in life.

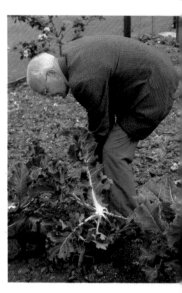

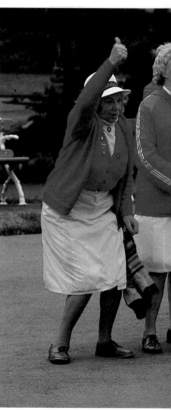

Top right: *It is important to stay active as you grow older, but since you have more time you can slow down a little.*
Right: *An element of competition is as valuable in the later years as it is earlier in life. It keeps you alert as well as active.*

As you get older, sports carry a greater risk of injury. However, a group of 200 runners over the age of 70 were able to avoid almost all trouble by sticking to a programme of gently performed stretching exercises (see page 26).

KEEPING FIT AFTER RETIREMENT

● Retirement is a time for relaxation without the stresses and strains of work, but it is a mistake to 'take things easy' in a physical sense. The ideal is to try and be even fitter physically than you were before retirement.

● With a little more time on your hands you should aim to be doing some sort of physical exercise for a least an hour every day.

● It is important to find some sort of activity that you enjoy. The core activities, especially walking, cycling and swimming, are just as appropriate in your sixties as in your thirties.

● It isn't necessary to push yourself hard physically all the time. The idea is to keep your body moving, and to keep the heart and lungs working a little harder than they do at rest. Activities such as gardening, ballroom dancing and bowls are more than sufficient. They are enough to keep the aerobic system working well, and they certainly help to keep you supple, even though they do not have the training effect needed to keep a competitive athlete in trim.

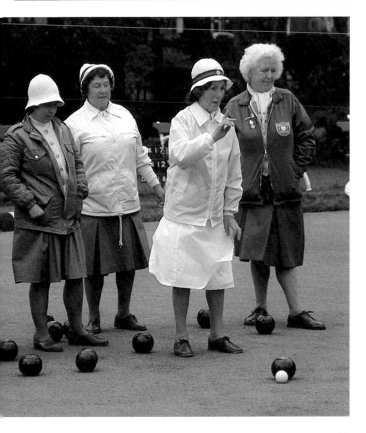

SPECIAL PROBLEMS ————————

So far in this book we have confined our attention to people who are completely healthy and wish to stay that way. Unfortunately everybody isn't completely healthy, and this bring up two questions:

● If you have some medical problem – such as asthma or diabetes – is there any reason why you shouldn't try to improve on your aerobic fitness?

● Does aerobic fitness actually help your medical problem?

Clearly the answers to these two questions will be influenced by the severity of the problem. A severe asthmatic, for example, may find it impossible to run more than a few steps. The advice given here is intended for people with mild or moderate disorders.

Diabetes controlled by insulin is no bar to strenuous exercise – in fact exercise is encouraged by diabetes specialists. Exercise does burn up extra fuel in the form of sugar, though, so diabetics on insulin may need extra food before a spell of exertion. Since most diabetics inject insulin into the legs and most sport involves the legs, more insulin may be released than usual – another reason why extra food may be needed.

Below: *Gary Mabutt has not allowed diabetes to keep him out of first-class football.*

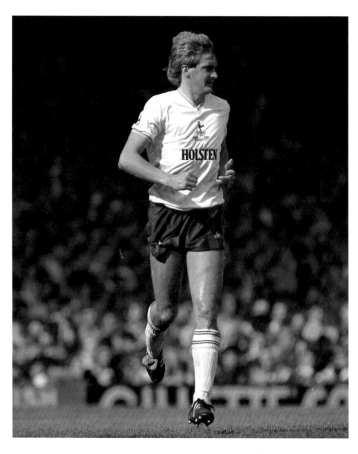

Asthma

Asthma isn't a bar to aerobic training unless it is quite severe. Many top class sportsmen and women suffer from mild degrees of asthma.

If you are a mild asthmatic, you may be perfectly fit in terms of your everyday activity, but you may start to wheeze and get into trouble as soon as you start pushing yourself. To some extent this can be helped by careful manipulation of your medication. It may be that some extra inhaled bronchodilators (the aerosols which widen the narrowed bronchial tubes) before you start out may help – this is obviously something to ask your doctor about.

Even with no change in your medication there are ways to get over the problem. It may be worth trying swimming – many sufferers find it less likely to provoke wheezing than, for example, running. If you do want to run or cycle, though, the thing to do is start off slowly and warm up slowly. If you feel a bit of a wheeze coming on, ease off a little – you will find that you can work up speed again later.

Bronchitis

Bronchitis comes on later in life, and here again the problem usually gets worse during exertion. This makes any aerobic training very hard, but there is some evidence that getting aerobically fitter does help.

Diabetes

For practical purposes diabetes can be divided into two separate conditions. About a tenth of diabetics develop their problem young (less than 30 years old) and need insulin from the start. The remainder develop diabetes later in life. This may be controlled by a special diet or tablets, but some sufferers need insulin.

For young diabetics, exercise is to be encouraged. There are many diabetic sportsmen, and quite a number of diabetics have run marathons. By careful manipulation of insulin and diet it is possible to do ultra-long-distance races, but this requires close collaboration between the diabetic and his advisers.

For older diabetics, aerobic training helps control the condition. If you are on insulin, however, you should seek medical advice. Even if you are on tablets you should tell your doctor you are starting to exercise more.

High blood pressure

High blood pressure is another condition on which exercise seems to have a beneficial effect, but caution is essential. The problem is that high blood pressure is one of the conditions that leads on to heart disease, and people who are likely to have heart disease are at the greatest risk of running into problems if they start to exercise (see page 32). If you have raised blood pressure you have to weight up the various risks before setting out on an intensive fitness regime, and this is something that has to be discussed with a doctor. Another aspect of this problem is that some of the drugs used to treat high blood pressure will reduce your capacity for strenuous exercise.

Angina and heart attacks

If you suffer from angina or have had a heart attack, energetic exercise may be risky. On the other hand it has been suggested that prudent physical training may improve both these conditions, and it is common for hospitals to provide supervised training programmes for heart attack patients, the main aim being to increase their self-confidence. As far as risk is concerned, there is little difference between people with angina, and people who have recently suffered heart attacks. The possible dangers depend very much on the extent of the problem, and medical advice is essential before embarking on an exercise programme of any kind.

SPORTS AND ACTIVITIES

Racket games

Racket games are among the most popular recreational activities these days. Interest in tennis has increased steadily with the growth of professional tennis, and the sport has long since ceased to be the prerogative of members of country clubs and owners of tennis courts. Enthusiasm for squash and badminton has grown at the same rate.

Given their undoubted popularity, how effective are they as forms of exercise? The players' skill is certainly an important factor, but this probably applies more to tennis than to other games such as squash and badminton. Unskilled tennis players simply lack the ability to expend very much energy in a useful way; this soon leads to a situation where they use the same amount of energy playing tennis as they would in brisk walking.

A more serious criticism of racket games is that they involve a high proportion of anaerobic exercise. You may think you have been running for hours on a squash court, but what has actually happened is that you have made a long series of short sprints, which have little or no aerobic training effect. In some cases aerobic fitness may do more for your squash than squash does for your fitness.

Racket games seem strenuous, but in a half-hour game, squash players are only actually in play for 15 minutes. This figure falls to 10 minutes for badminton and 5 minutes for tennis.

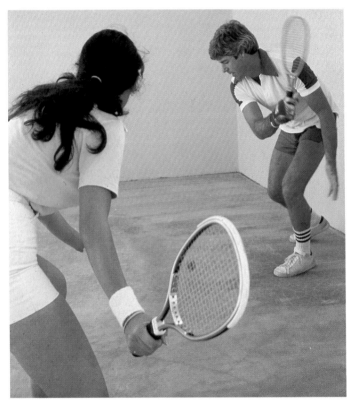

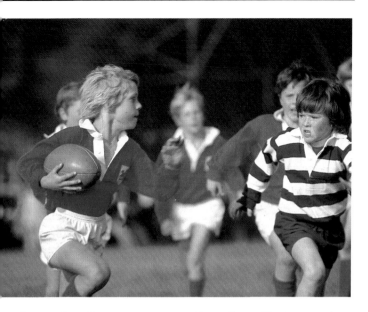

A note of caution

There has been mounting concern in the medical profession at the number of sudden deaths which occur on the squash court amongst older men. It is assumed that the explosive nature of the game precipitates heart problems in players who have heart disease. You should give up squash if you are known to have heart disease, and it is unwise for men to take up the game after the age of 40 even if they are fit.

Team sports

Participation in team sports such as soccer, hockey and rugby is the main reason why many people get fit and stay fit. These large-scale sports combine a high level of aerobic training with considerable mental interest and the spur of competition. Furthermore a game such as soccer requires very little in the way of specialised equipment; although it needs a pitch and two goal posts if it is to be played properly, we all know that it can be played almost anywhere with a ball, a bit of space and two old coats to act as a goal. It is also one of the most inter-

Above: Competitive team sports such as rugby and soccer are very effective at getting children really enthusiastic about physical exercise.

national of games. The only problem with such sports is the amount of physical contact they involve; this inevitably increases the risk of injury.

There are also a number of excellent team court games such as volleyball, netball, basketball and handball. These can be equally effective, but as the scale of the game becomes smaller there is a tendency for the exercise to become more anaerobic than aerobic (see Racket Games).

Although team games in general are a valuable aid to fitness, the fact that a game is played by a team does not necessarily mean that it provides good aerobic exercise. The classic example is cricket, in which only a few members of the team become involved in really strenuous activity. The rest would be much better off at home digging the garden so far as aerobic training is concerned.

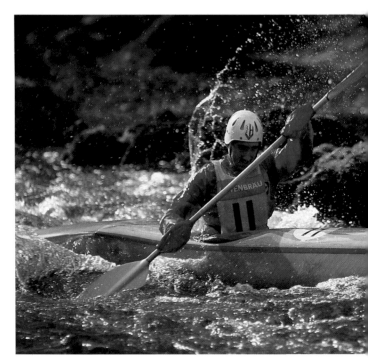

With the exception of swimming, we have not so far mentioned the huge range of activities that take place on (and in) the open water of lakes and the sea. Thousands of people participate in water sports and gain a lot of enjoyment along with their aerobic training. The convenience of these sports naturally depends on where you live, but it is surprising how much open water is available for recreational purposes even in the most land-locked parts of South Africa, for example, the Vaal Dam.

Canoeing
There are a variety of canoeing styles ranging from leisurely river touring to racing and battling with white water. Canoeing is excellent aerobic exercise and it is unique in being the only sport where a high degree of aerobic activity is demanded of the upper body rather than the legs.

Like all water sports safety has

Above: White water canoeing is particularly valuable exercise because most of the effort is put in by the shoulders and arms. In most sports the legs do the work. Right: Surfing is aerobically demanding because it depends on balance – and therefore hard work by the big postural muscles. Few sports are so exhilarating.

to be the paramount consideration – drowning is the major cause of recreational fatalities in most developed countries. For this reason, if for no other, expert teaching is desirable.

Rowing
Competitive rowing has a very large following in many countries, and is very good exercise. Although it may look to the uninitiated as though the bulk of the work is done with the arms, this is not the case. The art lies in transferring the power of the back and leg muscles out to the end of the oar.

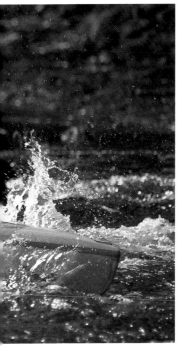

It is among the most intensively aerobic of sports, but like canoeing it is highly skilled, and expert tuition is essential. Because of the strain imposed on the back, especially if the rower uses faulty technique, it is not a sport to be taken up after the age of 35.

Sailing
Sailing can range from sitting in the cockpit of an offshore cruiser in a light wind, which has no aerobic value at all, to hanging out on the end of the trapeze of a racing dinghy in a force five wind – which has a lot. Consequently the value of sailing as a form of aerobic training varies considerably. As a general rule the smaller the boat, the more energetic the sailing.

The sport needs experience and expert teaching, but there are so many expert sailors around that teaching does not have to be professional. The sport varies in expense depending upon the boat involved.

Windsurfing
Windsurfing – or boardsailing – is a comparative newcomer to the scene. The sport depends upon the modern technology that enables the mast to be attached to the board by a strong universal joint. In all but the lightest winds it is highly aerobic since it depends upon balance, and therefore involves a good deal of work by the postural muscles. On average it is cheaper than dinghy sailing and it does not need such large stretches of water.

Water skiing
This is another skilled activity which requires tuition. It may appear that the work is being done by the boat, but it is not so – the load borne by the legs and other postural muscles is so high that it becomes a quite intensive aerobic activity. As with any water sport safety is a major consideration, and it is undeniably an expensive pastime.

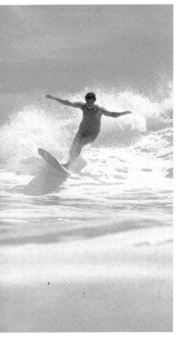

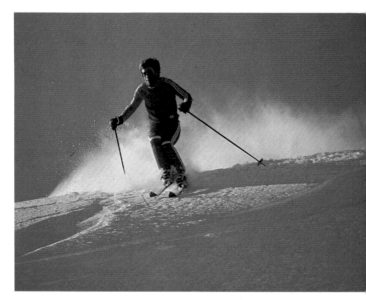

In sunny countries the winter does not cause such a problem as in colder countries. In some countries people can even swim throughout the year! Bad weather can, however, keep people indoors, and different ways of keeping fit must therefore be considered.

Apart from team sports like rugby and hockey, there are various other activities from which you could choose. You can attend aerobic classes throughout the year and gymnasiums are also available to those who take fitness seriously.

There is no reason whatsoever to become unfit during the winter months. A person who is only active in summer, struggles to regain his fitness after winter – and when he eventually succeeds at the end of summer, he looses it again.

Fitness is not like a sun-tan that you only get in summer. It is a way of life that continues even when the weather changes.

Skiing

Those who can go overseas for a skiing holiday or who can get to the few accessible ski resorts, do get plenty of exercise, especially if they make a considerable effort to

Above: *Downhill skiing has become immensely popular, and is very good exercise, but few people can afford to do it regulary.*

get fit *before* going skiing. The whole body benefits from this sport. Those who grab a pair of skis even though they are unfit usually end up having lots of fun, bruises and even injuries – without getting much exercise.

Skating

Indoor ice-rinks have made skating available to many people all the year round. It can be a very aerobic sport, but it requires skill and room on the ice if it is to be part of an intensive training regime.

Speed skating is a popular outdoor sport in countries with reliably freezing winters. It is a highly aerobic activity.

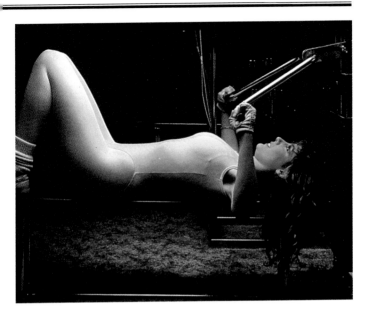

Above: *Gymnasiums offer a solution to those who want to remain fit during the winter.*

Below: *Skating is the only winter sport which is always available. Pursued energetically, it can have a valuable training effect.*

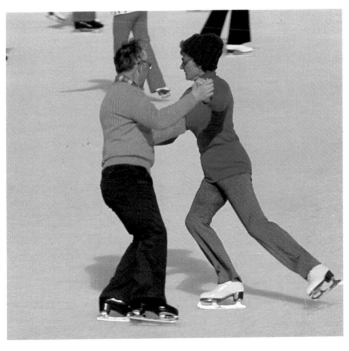

Riding

Riding horses does not at first appear to be a very strenuous activity, since the basic principle is that the horse does most of the work. However, riding depends on balance, which involves considerable exertion by the large postural muscles of the back, buttocks and legs. As a result of this, riding does have a useful training effect, although it is not as great as other balance-orientated sports such as downhill skiing, windsurfing or water skiing.

What applies to riding horses also applies to motorcycling, particularly in cross-country events such as scrambles and trials. While these are not among the most aerobic of activities, they do have some training value.

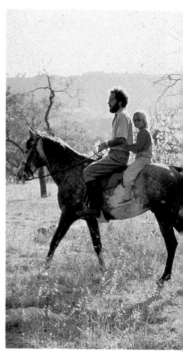

Golf

A round of golf involves a walk of about 8 km on average, but this is taken at different speeds by different players; what with waiting for your opponent to play, and fitting in with the other players on the course, the pace could hardly be described as brisk. The actual business of golf – hitting the ball – constitutes very short episodes of very anaerobic exercise which only serve to interrupt any aerobic training that is going on.

Golf is an excellent form of relaxation which is quite properly enjoyed by millions of people around the world, but because it is described as a 'sport' people naturally assume that it is 'healthy'. This is certainly not so if by healthy they mean that it has a valuable aerobic training effect.

The same applies to other 'healthy outdoor activities' such as fishing and shooting. These depend on the amount of time spent walking for their aerobic training value.

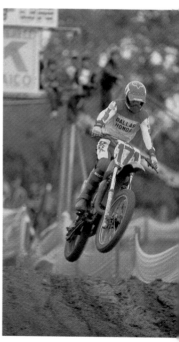

Back to walking

So we come back to walking – one of the most basic of human activities. The rate of energy

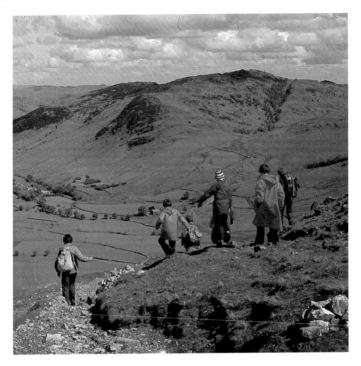

Top left: *Riding a horse at a gentle pace is very relaxing, but hard riding can be a quite demanding activity.*
Left: *Cross-country motorcycling depends on balance, which exercises the big muscles of the back and legs.*
Above: *Walking is the simplest form of aerobic exercise – but also one of the best.*

expenditure is not as high when you are walking as when you are running, swimming or cycling flat out. Fast swimming burns up three times as many kilojoules every minute as fast walking. However, many people would rightly regard a trip to the pool and a 20-minute swim as adequate exercise for the day. When people make a deliberate effort to go out walking, they will usually devote a fair amount of time to it, and to burn up the same amount of energy and benefit from the same total training effect, you only have to be walking for one hour – a walk of about 8 km at a brisk pace.

Orienteering

Map reading is the basis of one of the most intriguing sports to have emerged over the course of the last ten years – the sport of orienteering. The object is a simple one: to find your way from check-point to check-point over a piece of country you haven't seen before. Competitors are timed, and the fastest time wins, but you are not usually racing alongside your opponents.

Most orienteers do the course at a run, but running speed isn't everything. A brisk walker who can find his way accurately will do better than a fast runner who can't read a map. The sport combines the excitement of problem solving using map and compass with the spur of competition, and supplies a powerful motive for keeping fit.

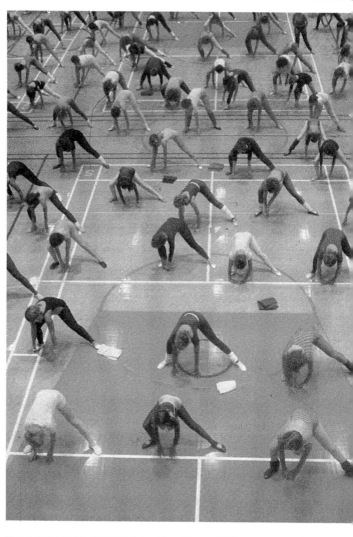

There have been countless studies aiming to show that aerobic exercise on its own reduces the risk of further problems after a heart attack. While this has never been convincingly demonstrated it has been shown that supervised physical training reduces the risk of depression and improves the chances of getting back to work quickly.

Above: While many sports have a valuable training effect it is the core activities such as aerobics which are most efficient at developing all-round fitness. Right: This chart shows how the various sports and activities rate as means of developing stamina, strength and flexiblity – the three main aspects of fitness. Stamina is the most important for general health, but flexibility and strength are both valuable assets.

Activities	Stamina	Strength	Flexibility
digging	☆☆	☆☆	☆☆
climbing stairs	☆☆☆	☆☆	☆☆
running	☆☆☆☆	☆☆☆	☆
aerobics	☆☆☆	☆☆	☆☆☆☆
swimming	☆☆☆☆	☆☆☆☆	☆☆☆
cycling	☆☆☆☆	☆☆☆	☆☆
keep-fit machines	☆☆☆	☆☆☆	☆☆
tennis	☆☆	☆☆	☆☆
squash	☆☆	☆☆☆	☆☆☆
badminton	☆☆	☆☆	☆☆
soccer	☆☆	☆☆☆	☆☆
hockey	☆☆	☆☆	☆☆
rugby	☆☆	☆☆☆	☆
volleyball	☆☆☆	☆☆	☆☆☆
netball	☆☆	☆☆	☆☆
basketball	☆☆☆	☆☆	☆☆
handball	☆☆☆	☆☆	☆☆☆
cricket	☆	☆	☆☆
canoeing	☆☆☆	☆☆☆	☆☆
rowing	☆☆☆☆	☆☆☆☆	☆
sailing (cruisers)	☆	☆☆	☆
sailing (dinghies)	☆☆	☆☆	☆☆
windsurfing	☆☆☆	☆☆☆	☆☆
water skiing	☆☆	☆☆☆	☆
cross-country skiing	☆☆☆☆	☆☆☆	☆☆☆
downhill skiing	☆☆	☆☆☆	☆☆☆
skating	☆☆	☆☆	☆☆☆
speed skating	☆☆☆	☆☆☆	☆☆
horse riding	☆	☆☆☆	☆
motorcycling (trials)	☆☆	☆☆☆	☆
golf	☆☆	☆	☆☆
fishing	☆	☆	☆
shooting (rough)	☆☆	☆	☆
shooting (target)	☆	☆	☆
walking (distance)	☆☆	☆	☆
orienteering	☆☆☆	☆☆☆	☆

PICTURE CREDITS

Artists Copyright of the artwork illustrations on the pages following the artists' names is the property of Salamander Books Ltd.
Milne Stebbing Illustration: 13, 15, 16, 17, 20, 22, 23, 24, 25, 26, 27, 41, 48, 49, 50, 51, 52.

Photographs The publishers wish to thank the following photographers and agencies who have supplied photographs for this book. The photographs have been credited by page number and position on the page: (B) bottom, (T) Top, (BL) Bottom Left etc.
Ace Photo Agency: (A.P. Turney) 23(T), (D. Bunce) 43, 70
All-Sport: 28, (Trevor Jones) 34, 64
Cannons Sports Club (UK) Ltd: 10/11(T)
Sally & Richard Greenhill: 10(BL), 12(T), 29, 37(T), 38, 39, 44, 56(TR), 56(BR), 58(T), 60/61, 62, 62/63(B), 73(T)
The Image Bank: (Elyse Lewin) 8/9(B), (Fulvio Roiter) 9(TR), (Zao Longfield) 14(B), (Michael Salas) 21, (John Kelly) 72(B), (J. Dimaggio/J. Kalish) 33(C), (N. Mareschal) 42, (Norbert Schafer) 54/55(B), 74(T), (The Production Co.) 57, (Burton McNeely) 68/69 (T), (Douglas J. Fisher) 71 (T)
New Health Magazine: 12(B), 18, 40, 66
The Photographers' Library:
Rex Features: 46/47
Spectrum Colour Library: 20(T)
Tony Stone Photolibrary-London: Endpapers, 30/31, 37(B), 45, 48(T), 53(B), 59(T), 69, 71(B)
Transworld Features: (Nicholas Tikhomiroff/Parents) Title page, (Enfants) 6, (Parents) 55(T)
Zefa: 26(T), 52(B), 72(T), Front Cover, Back cover

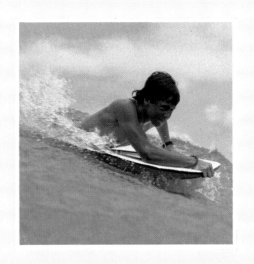

PRINTED IN BELGIUM BY
proost
INTERNATIONAL BOOK PRODUCTION